A Vision of Exercise

Tales of Inspiring People and Organisations

Andrew Edwards

Oakamoor
Publishing

Published by Oakamoor Publishing, an imprint of Bennion Kearny Limited
6 Woodside
Churnet View Road
Oakamoor
Staffordshire
ST10 3AE

www.BennionKearny.com

Table of Contents

Foreword

Mental health was something unbeknown to me growing up. I had no knowledge of what it meant, how it affected someone, and what effect it had on others. But if I look back, the signs were so obvious. Avoidance was my greatest weapon, steering clear of social occasions using training or sport as an excuse.

My first real indication was when I returned to my prep school for the evening to hand out awards. A winner dipped for me, so I could place the medal over his head, only for his face to return to me as a blur. My heart was pounding; I became hot and faint. Panic set in for fear of embarrassment. I tried to gather myself for the next winner, but I was on my way to what I now know as an anxiety attack. I reverted back to what I knew best… an excuse. I promptly made up a story and off I went in search of fresh air and a moment alone.

I left the school ashamed and embarrassed, gaining a memory and a feeling that sticks with me to this day. I didn't know what it was, and the fear of a repeat episode still haunts me now. But why did it happen to me?

I struggled with all of this for six years and kept it all to myself. In the beginning, I had rare episodes around public speaking and interviews but put it down to nerves. I assumed it was normal and refused any prospect of illness. My cricket remained largely untouched until I gained expectation; from media, fans, teammates, coaches, myself. I recall running off to vomit out of worry that I wouldn't be successful for my country; the anxiety was well and truly embedded in the game I adored. A World Cup was looming and having just reached no.1 in the world; I had to be the best, I had to prove the ranking was justified. I could not fail. I strongly believe everyone in sport has a fear of failure, to an extent. For some, it can help you thrive, but for others, it can be debilitating. Mine was the latter.

When the 2016 T20 World Cup in India arrived, I had failed before I got on the plane, and declared myself a failure as it was easier to deal with that than the pressure and worry of being unsuccessful. I would lay awake at night thinking about everything that could go wrong and did. The tournament gave me an average of less than 10, an attack before most games, and the need to be away from people and stuck in my room. My closest teammates and the coaching staff realised something was wrong; they all asked if I was alright, but I didn't have a clue what was going on. I just knew I didn't want to leave my room or play cricket again. Anxiety had won.

My lack of awareness about anxiety and a fear of being vulnerable led me to bottle every negative thought I ever had and, at some point, I had to implode. Luckily for me, the right person came into my life at the right moment, Mark Robinson, our head coach. For the first time, it was made ok for me to be vulnerable and express my feelings without fear of consequence. Between us, we knew – for the sake of my health – that I had to walk away from the game.

My break was indefinite and, for a time, my condition worsened – so much so that I was unable to leave my bed. For months, I only left the house for a moment, reaching 200 metres before panic set in and I'd have to return home. As well as dealing with this, I had lost purpose in life; I found no reason to actually get up in the morning. No drive.

It took me seven months to build up the courage to consider picking up a bat. In that time, I saw a clinical psychologist who helped me learn about mental health and anxiety. What it was, why I had it, and what could be done. My anxiety wasn't because of cricket, it was everything in between. I had let negativity and worry consume me, as in my mind, failure was bad, no matter what I was doing.

Re-joining the squad was a gradual build-up over six months; my anxiety had to be tested, but at a pace that was comfortable for me, along with low expectations as to the level I should be performing at. The more I joined in, the more confident I became. Joining fitness sessions was a major concern for me. I had always been fit, but I'd had a year out. With this, it meant I worried at looking unfit or not completing a running session, especially in front of the girls. A quick tap on the shoulder and a reminder that I should have low expectations helped me push through my fears, and I am now fitter than I ever have been. Fitness and exercise are now in my life every day.

The nature of cricket brings more failure than most. A sport with plentiful moments of isolation to allow for overthinking and doubt. On the international stage, critics are ready to jump on a mistake, and with social media at the end of your fingertips, it's hard to escape. But with the right team environment and people around you, it can go a long way in removing all of the above concerns.

I was lucky enough to return to an environment that was one of praise for putting yourself out there and failing, one where saying you're vulnerable was encouraged. How can failure be praised? Why would admitting your vulnerabilities be a good thing? I know now. Sharing your struggles is no weakness. Owning up to any worry is a strength. How else do you learn? The girls embraced my worries, opened up about their own, and made me see I am not alone. We are all in it together. And we were all there, together, a year later, lifting that World Cup at Lord's against India against the odds. A place I thought I would never be.

My anxiety is a part of me, but no longer rules my life. The constant battles are lessening, and anxiety is no longer winning. I have strategies in place that the whole team have kindly bought into, and I have thrived, bounding over every hurdle put in my way. Speaking out was the first step to my recovery, and the more people that do will help others realise it doesn't make you weak. It takes a strong individual to stand up and fight, and that will only come with knowledge. Ignorance is not bliss in this instance; raised awareness and knowledge of mental health is important for all, not just the ones who suffer.

The combination of endorphins released after running, and the achievement of getting through a hard session in front of the team, empowers me to tackle my anxiety. I walk away with the mindset of, "If I can get through that, then I can get through anything." I have conquered major anxiety hurdles after training, and I have no doubt in my mind there's a correlation.

Therefore, I applaud all the contributors to this book and greatly respect Andrew for his bravery on speaking out in detail about his own battles regarding mental health and managing his autism on a daily basis. A person we could all learn plenty from.

Sarah Taylor

England, Sussex, and Surrey Stars Bat/Wicket-keeper | Four-time Ashes Winner | Three-time World Cup Winner

Prologue

Exercise is considered vital for maintaining physical and mental fitness. It can be effective at improving alertness, concentration, and cognitive function, and can be especially helpful when stress has depleted a person's energy or ability to concentrate. When stress affects the brain, with its many nerve connections, the rest of the body feels the impact as well. Conversely, if your body feels better, so does your mind.

Scientists have found that regular participation in aerobic exercise can decrease overall levels of tension, and elevate and stabilize mood, improve sleep, and enhance self-esteem. The National Health Service prescribes exercise to deal with some cases of depression and anxiety, and a study in the U.S.A. has shown that by increasing your activity levels from nothing to exercising at least three times a week you can reduce your risk of depression by almost 20%.

So, with the benefits of exercise clear for all to see, I would like to share the stories of people who have overcome personal challenges thanks to the power of exercise, and organisations and individuals which have worked hard to have a positive effect on those with disabilities.

Over the course of this book, I want to show the positive effect that exercise can have on anyone's life; from mine to others with disabilities (both physical and mental) or disadvantage. I have experienced the effects of exercise and I want to see it from others' perspectives. Let's get started!

1. Sabrina Fortune

Whilst training in July 2017, my coach and trainer – Geraint – told me about a Paralympic medallist who he also trained at the gym three days a week. That Paralympian was Wrexham-born, Flintshire-raised, 20-year-old F20 shot putter Sabrina Fortune. The F20 category is for athletes with an intellectual impairment who compete in throwing events; in Sabrina's case Speech Dyspraxia.

Speech Dyspraxia, also known as Development Verbal Dyspraxia, is a condition where the individual is unable to fully offer sounds, syllables, and words. It is caused by a separation between the brain and the speech muscles where co-ordination gets lost; the cause is unknown, and there is no known cure.

Whilst viewing Twitter footage of Sabrina deadlifting 105kg, which was a personal best for her, at my gym, I heard a familiar voice in the background. It was Geraint. He made the introductions in the real-world, and I asked Sabrina to elaborate on how her coaches have helped her (like they have with me and my autism) in achieving her goals.

"Ed [Harper], Geraint [Roberts] and all the guys in the Number One gym have been amazing. I have lost over a stone so far this year with diet and exercise, and I am already stronger and fitter than I was. They have helped me a lot by gaining my trust and made me feel more confident. They help me a lot with my balance and strength and always make training fun. They always cheer me up."

With this in mind, I asked Sabrina, how she first got into training at age eleven.

"I got into training because my older brother had been training and competing in athletics and I wanted to join in and compete with him. My older brother was my hero as I watched him compete for many years and wanted to be like him. Beverley Jones was also one of my heroes after seeing her win her medals." (Queensferry-born Jones, who has Cerebral Palsy and previously trained with Sabrina, won a bronze medal at London 2012 in the F37 Discus throw.)

Since first competing at a national level at age 15, whilst attending Buckley Argoed High School around the time of London 2012 (initially as a discus thrower), Sabrina's aim was to make the Paralympics in Rio in 2016. Success was not long in waiting for Sabrina as, after changing disciplines to the shot put, she won a gold medal at the 2014 Paralympic

Schools Championship in Rio; a prelude to her aim of success at the Paralympics two years later.

A fourth-place finish was achieved by Sabrina at the 2015 Paralympic World Championships in Doha, Qatar, with a throw of 12.14 metres. The same fourth-place was achieved at the 2016 Paralympic European Championships in the run-up to Rio. Alongside her performance in Qatar the previous year, Sabrina was undoubtedly a firm contender for success in Rio in September 2016.

After achieving a personal best throw of 12.94 metres in Rio, Sabrina – who represents Deeside Athletic Club – took home the bronze medal. In the process, she became the first Welsh athlete on the podium during the 2016 Paralympics.

Following her great success and achievement in Rio, closer to home award wins and nominations came Sabrina's way. She took home both the 2016 Wrexham County Borough Disability, and Senior Sports Personality of the Year, trophies, as she also represents Wrexham Special Olympics Club. She was nominated for the Disability Sport Wales Award for the second year running in 2016.

Most recently in 2017, Sabrina finished sixth in the F20 Shot Putt at the World Paralympic Championships at the Olympic Stadium in Stratford, East London.

Proving herself to be a great competitor under pressure in high profile events, it seems clear that the routine, discipline, and mental and physical benefits of training for competitions has aided Sabrina in managing her Dyspraxia.

"Competition and training has helped me so much. When I first started out, I was very shy and never talked because of my speech dyspraxia, and I had no confidence. I always stayed with my mum. Now I have much more confidence and enjoy travelling and going away with the Team.

"Routine is extremely hard for me, but the more I do it, the easier it gets. The physical and mental side of things is extremely hard. I use picture cards to help me remember warm-ups and routine in competition. My coaches give me simple but repetitive instructions.

"I find failure very hard to deal with but have a good psychologist to help me focus on my goals. I have a nutritionist who helps me to eat the right foods at the right time."

I asked how Sabrina's condition had affected her.

"It has been very hard growing up with my disability. I got bullied and made fun of in school, as I was in mainstream education but in the language unit receiving intensive speech therapy. Sport has helped me gain confidence so much, and the hate I felt towards people who bullied me helps drive me forward in my sport."

Apart from training and competing, Sabrina attended Coleg Cambria in Deeside, where she started a two-year catering course. She now does Sugar Craft on a Monday and told me that, "I would love to own my own cake business one day."

Finally, I asked Sabrina for the best piece of advice she had received in either life or training.

"My advice would be to keep training fun and make the most of every opportunity – whether you're having a bad day or a good day. Always be kind to other people. Let people know you for your ability not your disability. Don't let anyone tell you can't achieve because you can! I did it and so can you. Never give up keep chasing your dream and make it happen because, when it does, it is truly amazing."

2. Rochdale Mind

As a legacy of London 2012, Sport England has seen participation figures in core Olympic sports such as swimming, cycling, and running, increase. Reasons include the freedom they offer in our schedule-stretched modern world, the little or no travel required, the lack of equipment needed, and (often) the sport being self-sufficient (i.e., no team needed). Historically popular sports such as cricket, golf, and eleven-a-side football have seen declining numbers, although five- and seven-a-side and walking football have seen increased participation.

Seeking to get more people taking part in sport and exercise, to the betterment of their physical and mental wellbeing, The *Get Set to Go* initiative was launched in July 2015 – by the mental health charity *Mind* – and aims to improve the lives of people with mental health problems through access to physical activity and sport in their local communities. The programme seeks to remove the barriers that people living with mental health issues often face.

After finding out about the Get Set to Go programme, which is supported by Sport England and The National Lottery, I travelled to Rochdale in Greater Manchester to learn more. Rochdale and District Mind were selected alongside health services in Croydon, Middlesbrough & Stockton-on-Tees, Tyneside & Northumberland, Dudley in the West Midlands, Herefordshire, other areas of Lancashire, and Brent in North West London.

After bidding for funding, Rochdale was chosen along with the other seven areas in the pilot scheme because of high inactivity in the local population and because they are one of the poorest areas in England. This is said to be a legacy of the town's hitherto reliance on the prosperity of being a mill town.

Regarding inactivity, a 2012 Health Survey for England found that people today are far less active than in the past. This has serious implications for our physical and mental health. The survey found that just 67% of men and 55% of women, aged 16 years and over, meet the recommended 150 minutes of activity per week.

So, in September 2016, I met up with Melanie Tilley – Mind's coordinator – and within minutes of engaging in conversation with her, I found her enthusiasm and passion for her work to be infectious. I also found learning about Get Set to Go's aims and experiences, and what many of their service users experienced, to be similar to what I had encountered in my life. For you see, when I suffered from clinical depression between early 2011 and April 2014, exercise was one of the few times I felt comfortable in my life.

To attend a session, people must be aged 16 or over and living with, or showing, symptoms of a mental health problem. Individuals can join without receiving treatment whilst also not requiring a GP's referral. Taster sessions are available, and there is no obligation to participate further in future activities.

The aims of the Get Set to Go Physical Activity / Sports programme are to:

- Provide the opportunity for people to try out a variety of different sports / physical activities
- Encourage people to discover the physical and mental well-being benefits that come from taking part in exercise
- Offer the chance to meet and connect with new people within Rochdale and District Mind, and within community sports provider organisations
- Provide the opportunity to learn new skills
- Encourage people to engage in social activities
- Reduce isolation

In the local gyms in Rochdale, Melanie works closely with local sport and recreation providers. Staff, ranging from receptionists to instructors, are trained to deal with service users and people with mental health problems generally. One example occurred when a trainer guided a new service user to GStG's meeting point at the local gym after the receptionist forgot to inform them where GStG meets up. Without the understanding of the trainer, this service user may have been put off attending future sessions.

Melanie also told me of an instance when a trainer failed to pick up on a service user's negative body language at a session. The individual was initially put off attending again, until Melanie went to the next session to help develop their confidence. Due to her positive intervention, the service user continues to attend activities.

From January 2016, the training given to local sport and recreation providers in Rochdale has been free of cost, although some activities have a small subsidized fee for service users depending on the provider, so they feel more comfortable welcoming people with mental health issues to sessions. Hopefully, this snapshot further reinforces the positive steps made in the gyms with people with mental health issues.

Many of GStG's instructors are volunteers, some of whom had taken an interest in sport and exercise after becoming service users of GStG. In Rochdale, there are 12 volunteers in total, ranging in age from 21 to 63. The team of volunteers provide support to people attending sporting activities either on a one-to-one basis or as part of a team or group.

Melanie explained how previous mental health sufferers often had little confidence but had gone on to be volunteers after gaining self-worth and self-esteem from physical activity; they also took the lessons and skills learnt exercising into other aspects of their lives, whilst the social aspect of GStG was greatly beneficial.

Unfortunately, there seems to be reticence from local GPs in terms of referring patients, although when I met Melanie, she did have a future meeting with a number of local doctors regarding the matter. So, as I write, hopefully much progress has been made. To me, it is surprising that GPs are not making referrals as you hear (almost daily) stories in the media from medical professionals espousing the virtues of regular physical activity in order to prevent all sorts of conditions, illnesses, and ailments.

The following table details the wide variety of sports available in Rochdale and the numbers of people being referred and engaged over three months.

ACTIVITY	REFERRED	ENGAGED	NO OF SESSIONS
Archery	21	19	2
Badminton Middleton	1	1	4
Badminton Rochdale	4	2	12
Boxing	6	3	9
Canoeing	0	0	0
Climbing	1	0	0
Cycling	4	4	9
Football	4	4	13
Gym Heywood	0	0	0
Gym Middleton	3	3	15
Gym Rochdale	8	6	21

ACTIVITY	REFERRED	ENGAGED	NO OF SESSIONS
Independent Activities	N/A	N/A	N/A
Kayaking – see canoeing			
Mindfulness Ramble	5	4	3
Pilates	2	1	12
Rambling Middleton	0	0	2
Rambling Rochdale	8	4	11
Running	1	0	0
Swimming Heywood	0	0	12
Swimming Middleton	2	2	1
Swimming Rochdale	4	1	11
Tai Chi Heywood	0	0	0
Tai Chi Rochdale	3	1	7
Yoga	0	0	0
Youth Gym	0	0	0
Zumba Heywood	0	0	3
Zumba Middleton	0	0	0
TOTALS	77	55	147

- Over the last quarter of 2016, there was a total of 16 different physical activities taking place – 12 taking place on a weekly basis with badminton in Middleton fortnightly. Gym sessions in Middleton and Rochdale were twice weekly, and so was archery.

- There were two new GStG activities between Oct and Dec 2016

- 105 participants have taken part in GStG activities over Q4 2016 (274 participants since the project started)

- There were 654 GStG activity attendances over Q4 2016 (3841 attendances since the project started)

- 57 non-Mind clients have attended activities between October and December 2016 (350 since the project started)

- The Lancashire FA and Rochdale F.C. finally become involved with the football group. The Lancashire FA has provided them with new kit and has given them equipment. Rochdale F.C., meanwhile, provided a coach early in 2017.

- There was a group of about 6-8 people that play badminton every Saturday independently of GStG and who attended gym and swimming outside of GSTG groups using L4L cards

The final statistics for Get Set to Go from the report evaluation summary were:

- Nationwide, 3,585 people with mental health issues have taken part in the project

- The evaluation teams from Loughborough and Northampton Universities tracked 1,000 Get Set To Go participants making it the "largest study of its kind internationally"

- On average, participants increased activity levels by 1.3 days a week

- 76% rated the programme as very good or excellent after three months with that number rising to 78% after six months

- 80% of participants were very or fairly satisfied with the programme at three months, and 86% of participants were very or fairly satisfied at six months

The legacy for Get Set to Go includes:

- Mind in Camden have incorporated Get Set to Go into their Healthy Minds programme with support from local commissioners

- Middlesbrough and Stockton Mind have been commissioned to extend the model to Stockton, working closely with mainstream leisure providers to support people with mental health problems to become more physically active

- 25 local Minds have been licensed to deliver Mental Health Awareness for Sport and Physical Activity training across England and Wales

- The Exercise Referral Scheme Wales, and Sport Wales, commissioned Newport Mind to pilot Mental Health Awareness for Sport and Physical Activity training in five areas of Wales. Discussions around extending Get Set to Go into Wales are also taking place

- Along with the Sport and Recreation Alliance and the Professional Players Federation, Mind has supported over 280 signatories of the Mental Health Charter for Sport and Recreation. Mind is developing more resources to support the sector, and will be offering tailored training and consultancy

In my opinion, the Get Set to Go programme is an excellent example of helping people to change their lives for the better – emotionally, mentally and physically. I hope it can be the forerunner to more people with mental health issues benefiting from the many great aspects that exercise and sport participation can provide.

3. Brickfield Rangers

As a local resident who was born and bred with a big interest in Welsh Pyramid football, I have been aware of Brickfield Rangers Football Club for over 15 years and known several people who have turned out for the senior men's team over that period. I was also mildly aware of the club's many other teams, ranging from women, girls, and futsal, and their engagement with people in local villages for community cohesion, and help for the disabled.

Since Brickfield's formation by "enthusiastic" parents in 1976, it has become multi-award winning and counts Robbie Savage and Zambian born ex-Manchester City and Northern Ireland international players The Whitley Brothers amongst its junior section alumni in years gone by.

Brickfield Rangers is also approved by the U.K. branch Special Olympics, are founder members of the North Wales Disability League (which hold monthly tournaments for both youth and senior players), and hold a UEFA Fun Football License enabling them to meet the school curriculum fully.

Not just at Brickfield, but across Wales, disability football is thriving. In February 2004, Brickfield was the only disability club across the Principality. In 2015, this number had risen sharply to 30 clubs operating 60 teams with more than 800 players on the books.

I got in touch with Andrew Ruscoe, Brickfield's Director of Football, who is behind a great deal of this fantastic work and arranged a meeting with him at Wrexham County Museum. Within minutes of meeting Andrew, I was immediately struck by his sheer enthusiasm, determination, and drive to get his message and belief about how participating in football can be empowering. Andrew's message is that for every Wayne Rooney, Cristiano Ronaldo or Lionel Messi, there are hundreds of thousands of people from all different backgrounds, skill levels, and social, academic, and emotional abilities that can be turned on to play a sport; in this instance, football.

In Andrew's role, sport is all about participation, fun, enjoyment, and overcoming barriers such as social isolation, and mental disorders. In addition to this, listening to Andrew, the physical, mental, social and general benefits of being part of a team (for any sport) are not to be underestimated.

Andrew firmly believes in the participation element; for club matches, he believes performance-related coaching, with its results-driven emphasis, would knock back and put off many of the disabled players he has dealt with. Andrew saw first-hand, in a previous role at another organisation where the emphasis wasn't on participation, how social inclusion and mental wellbeing could be helped; he decided he wanted a different approach where false hopes were not created.

He explained that when disabled players come to training, and monthly matches, it is often the highlight of their week. He sees smiles from people who may otherwise have had little to look forward to as (like myself) support funding may have been cut or (unlike myself) they are left to fend for themselves in an unforgiving world.

Football gives people hope, self-worth, social inclusion, teamwork and social and emotional skills that – without Brickfield Disability Football – they may not have been fortunate to have.

Further proof of Andrew's message is that one club participant, when they first attended sessions, was said to have seldom spoken. Eventually, this turned into smiles and positive body language before they fully expressed themselves within the group. This is a story I can certainly relate to as when I first joined Cefn Druids (a football club based just outside Wrexham) training sessions in late 1999, I was simply a supporter and not a member of the team; as above, my body language and feelings would have been apparent – I was socially isolated in my youth and taught in a classroom on my own at school. Going to Druids helped me immensely, both socially and emotionally, whilst also building my confidence and maturity in various capacities.

There are around 400 players on the books of Brickfield with 60 volunteers supervising them. The club has 28 affiliated teams, including six teams for girls and women. An important part of the club's ethos is to help minimise anti-social behaviour, whilst boosting active citizenship and promoting community cohesion.

The club runs a programme that caters for youngsters with disabilities in 12 Special Educational Units within Wrexham County Borough and neighbouring areas. The aim, again, is to encourage participation in sport whilst attempting to improve peoples' social skills and improve their mental, emotional, and physical health.

Andrew, or "Chopper" to give him his nickname, coaches at a number of these units after he put his own money, and the support of Brickfield Rangers, into his work. He has gained a postgraduate degree in Youth and Community at Glyndwr University whilst securing his teaching qualification to help him further these projects in Wrexham, to create better opportunities for youngsters in the area.

Like Rochdale Mind, Andrew likes to keep the cost of these sessions low. He firmly believes that when people have bills to pay and money is often extremely stretched, the cost must be kept low or people won't turn up to sessions. They will then miss out on the benefits that physical activity obviously brings both mentally and physically.

Fortunately, Andrew's beliefs and positive message seem to be getting through as, in 2016, he won a Welsh National Award, along with Brickfield, for Community Club of the Year. Later in 2016 (November to be precise), Andrew was jointly awarded the Wrexham Sports Coach Award for his work with BRFC Football in the Community. He was also nominated for Senior Volunteer of the Year.

Andrew's success and hard work are not just restricted to disability football; five young girls from Brickfield Rangers Junior Girls team have recently been asked to go on trial at one of the biggest clubs in the country… Everton. This would probably not have materialised without Andrew visiting various schools encouraging young girls, aged four to 14, to take part in sessions at Brickfield's Clywedog Park site with help from Glyndwr University's Girls ADOR Project.

Brickfield Rangers really has developed an enviable reputation. It has a name for developing footballing talent for most sections of society, whether that is professional footballers, people with disabilities, women players, or even disadvantaged youngsters. Truly Brickfield Rangers is a "club for all."

4. Disability Cricket

As someone with a life-long disability, plus a keen (at times obsessional) level of interest in the sound of leather on willow, it seemed natural for me to explore cricket as part of this book.

My actual playing "career", if I'm delusional enough to call it that, equated to a three-ball duck, batting at number three for my local village, Gwersyllt, which is the same one Robbie Savage also hails from. I only played at Under 15 level, away to neighbouring Llay Welfare CC. On the only other time I was selected, a matter of weeks later, I refused to be a specialist fielder (bat number 11 and not bowl).

On the latter occasion, playing for Gwersyllt Under 15's at Marchwiel-Wrexham CC, who won the National Village Knockout at Lord's in 1980 and 1984, I went home in a strop. I later trained with Marchwiel-Wrexham hoping and failing (partly due to supporting Cefn Druids F.C.) to get into the second eleven under the watchful guise of legendary pre-apartheid South African Test batsman, the late, Eddie Barlow. He had previously been Bangladesh's coach upon their Test bow in autumn 2000 against India.

So, as you can tell by reading the above, I am more of a cricket watcher than player. I was a Lancashire CCC member from 2004-2016 and love attending England Tests at Lord's and Old Trafford. In fact, I haven't missed the Saturday of an Old Trafford Test since 1998.

Therefore, I was interested in finding out more about players with disabilities who are a lot more talented at the sport I love than me. After watching interviews with the England Pan-Disability team and management on ICC Cricket Monthly on Sky Sports during summer 2016, one person who piqued my interest was Ian Martin. His was a name that I had heard mentioned in dispatches in North Wales Cricket. Ironically, I later found out there are two Ian Martins from the same village of Mynydd Isa, near Mold, who are involved in cricket! Nonetheless, I contacted the correct Ian Martin, who is Head of Disability Cricket at the England and Wales Cricket Board, and the one I was looking for.

Mr Martin is an interesting and remarkable man, who served a spell in the Royal Navy from 1987-1994, including in the First Gulf War in the early 1990s. Unfortunately, he had to leave the Navy after he was diagnosed with the genetic condition Charcot-Marie-Tooth disease (CMT) – a condition which progressively damages his peripheral nerves. It means Ian has to use a power chair to get by in his daily work.

Ian's first involvement within Disability Cricket occurred in North East Wales in 2000. Ian has been working full-time in Disability Cricket administration since April 2004, when he took a pay cut from working for M&S to work first for Disability Sport Wales as a Development Officer, before joining the England and Wales Cricket Board in November 2007. In the latter role, Ian was the first full-time employee for the ECB solely responsible for developing Disability Cricket and thus shelved his plans of the time to move Down Under.

Ian is a multi-award winner for his work in Disability Cricket administration including winning the Welsh Sports Admin of the Year Prize in July 2006 and being named "People's Champion" by Trinity Mirror Newspapers in the same year. Ian's history proves to me, if I needed any convincing, that sport can enable people to overcome barriers irrespective of race, religion, gender, sexuality or disability, whilst making a positive impact on lives around the world.

During our meeting in Wrexham before Ian made his way to Edgbaston to ready the Visually Impaired Squad for the 2017 World Cup in India (where they reached the semi-final before losing to Pakistan in Bangalore), I asked him about the mental and physical positive benefits that sport and exercise can have on people. He told me that players from the Learning Disability Squad saw the biggest difference. Many of them, when on tour with England, were away from home for the first time and grew in confidence with the right support and, of course, thanks to playing a sport they love.

A typical week for Ian includes going to Lord's for weekly meetings with various figures of the ECB hierarchy including Chief Executive Tom Harrison and legendary former England captain, Andrew Strauss, who since May 2015 has been Director of Cricket of the board. Within these meetings, it is Ian's role to report to the board regarding the issues that may have arisen within the various disability squads.

Over the decade he has been at the ECB, he has seen funding for disability cricket increase significantly. Part of this is due to disability equality being more advanced in the U.K. in comparison to many other traditional cricketing nations.

On the field, the Learning Disability Team (in their infancy) lagged far behind rival nations such as Australia and South Africa. However, the turning point in their performances occurred around 2009 with performances showing a marked improvement which, in turn, led to extra funding.

In fact, during the Tri-Series with South Africa and Australia held at various club grounds in Cheshire, in July 2017, the England Learning Disability Team went undefeated in five 40-over One Day Internationals, including the final at Neston Cricket Club. They were also undefeated in four Twenty 20 matches against the tourists, including the final at Nantwich Cricket Club. All in all, nine matches unbeaten for the hosts.

The extra funding across the board for all the disability teams has seen greatly improved resources made available to the players. These added resources include the use of nutritionists, trainers, professionals who deal with mental and emotional aspects, dieticians, and analysts. All considered, it is rather comforting for someone with a disability to realise that they are afforded the use of a similar band of support staff to the likes of Joe Root, Alastair Cook, Ben Stokes, Jimmy Anderson, Stuart Broad, et al. Players have structured fitness programmes that help target weaknesses that need to be worked on. The fitness programmes entail the players train at least three times a week in their own time.

Rather understandably, Ian explained to me, given the investment involved both financially and professionally (in terms of time and expertise), if a player isn't performing to the expected standard and loses their place in the squad they, of course, lose ECB support.

Once players are established members in the team they tend to mainly appear for the national disability squad over other levels of cricket although, when National duty isn't calling, several players appear in the various ECB Premier Divisions around the country.

Interestingly, the Learning Disability captain, Chris Edwards, played for Caldy CC, against Nantwich Town CC in April 2015 when Lancashire and England batsman Liam Livingstone smashed an astonishing 350 not out for Nantwich Town CC off just 138 balls, in the 45 over match for the National Club Knockout Group Six, First Round match. Unfortunately for Chris Edwards, Caldy were then bowled out for just 79 as they lost by an overwhelming 500 run margin. Chris, however, did top score with 27 off 21 balls whilst opening the batting.

One very interesting story from the Physical Disability team revolves around 21-year-old Callum Flynn from Leigh, Lancashire. Callum was diagnosed with bone cancer on his 14th birthday and it resulted in him undergoing a life-saving operation. This was followed by five months of chemotherapy that left him wheelchair-bound at the time. In addition to this, Callum underwent two years of intensive physiotherapy and now has a titanium knee.

Not to be put off by this major setback at such a young age, Callum raised £50,000 for Bone Cancer Research. In 2011, this led to him being named "Britain's Kindest Kid" by The Charities Foundation. Callum has also campaigned for life-altering medication (Mephat) to be made available on the NHS.

At age 16, Callum made his debut for Lancashire CCC Disability Team. His disability cricket career has gone to such heights that he was a part of England's team that won the inaugural Physical Disabilities World Cup in Bangladesh in Autumn 2015. This helped him earn the 2016 England Disability Player of the Year Award at a ceremony that also saw Joe Root awarded Men's Player of the Year, Charlotte Edwards crowned Women's Player of the Year, and a lifetime achievement award bestowed upon Cricket's "Renaissance Man" – David "Bumble" Lloyd.

Away from cricket, Callum attended Myerscough College in Preston and now attends University of Central Lancashire on a Monday and Tuesday. He also turns out for Swinton Moorside CC in the Greater Manchester League in non-disability cricket.

Whilst Callum Flynn and Chris Edwards play for the Physical and Learning Disability squads respectively, the Visually Impaired team are categorized into three different sections. B1 Players are completely blind, B2s have restricted sight, and B3s are partially sighted.

The ball used for Visually Impaired players is a plastic ball containing ball bearings to aid their reactions to facing the delivery. The ball is delivered underarm and has to touch two sides of the wicket.

There is an enlightening video available online of England limited overs captain, Eoin Morgan, attempting to bat in the nets at his home ground of Lord's whilst wearing, at various times, three different glasses that replicate what visually impaired players wear out in the middle.

Firstly, Morgan wore the B3 (partially sighted) glasses which resulted in him being bowled twice in the first three deliveries he faced. It got no easier for him with the B2 (restricted sight) glasses as he got out leg before wicket. Finally, with the B1 (completely blind) glasses, Morgan played a sweep shot with significantly less conviction than in any of his One Day International innings.

So, after viewing Eoin Morgan trying to play with visually impaired goggles, I was extremely keen to learn more and try them on myself. A visit was arranged for Saturday 7th October 2017 at Edgbaston Cricket Ground, Birmingham, where the Visually Impaired Squad were meeting up to train for end of season physical and mental tests.

37-year-old Ross Hunter is England's coach for the visually impaired team and was appointed to his role in April 2013 replacing Chris Porter. In his playing career, he was based in Hampshire and reached England Under 17 level as a wicketkeeper-bat whilst also playing second eleven cricket for Derbyshire and Hampshire. In May 2017, he became the first full-time England Disability coach, along with ex-Sussex, Surrey and England Test leg-spinner Ian Salisbury who, along with his role with the Women's team, became the Physical Disability Coach.

After meeting Ross, I met with England's Team Manager for the visually impaired, Martin Dean. Martin was a very welcoming, talkative, amiable gentleman and has been in his manager's role since 2008. Indeed, Martin has been involved in coaching visually impaired cricket and football since the turn of the millennium. Martin, himself, has a condition called Usher Syndrome, which is "an extremely rare genetic disorder caused by a mutation in any one of at least eleven genes resulting in visual impairment and, in some cases deafness. It is at present, incurable."

Martin told me that today was the end of season tests that are used to gauge fitness and other targets set for the players at the beginning of the year. During this time, they are also set subsequent targets across the season.

Martin explained to me that there are many different related conditions on the visually impaired spectrum. Some visually impaired people may only have one condition, whereas others may have three or four totally different visual impairments. He passed me five types of visually impaired goggles, which represented five conditions: Macular Degeneration, Diabetic Retinopathy, Glaucoma, Cataract, and Blindness.

I tried on the five pairs of goggles for a brief move around. The first pair I tried on were the "blackout" goggles representing total blindness. I could not wear them for a long period of time and even then, I was moving very slowly with a total lack of direction. I also tried on the other goggles to get a feel for the different conditions.

Martin told me to expect my hearing to be sharper when wearing the "blackout" goggles when I batted. He also informed me that when the England Visually Impaired Team play sighted opposition, they ask members of the other team to try on a pair of "Tunnel Vision" goggles for "around ten or a dozen overs." Many of the sighted players, who have tried on the goggles have, according to Martin, had severe headaches. However, they are always informed of the risks attached beforehand and to immediately remove them if they have any issues arising from their use.

Whilst I was talking to Martin, I was intrigued by a mat session on the floor near the nets for the players who didn't have total blindness. The mat had eight different sections with four colours that consisted of red, blue, green and yellow. The mat had 36 sub-sections related to various aspects of performance, teamwork, and individual personality characteristics. The mat is called an Insight Mat, and its aim is offer an understanding into traits such as player personalities, decision making, and potential leadership skills. With the mat, players are asked to respond to certain theoretical scenarios that can help deduce mental and emotional skills in pressure situations. The session was led by Lara Barrett, Performance Psychologist, who as well as the England and Wales Cricket Board, works alongside Para Tri-athletes and Squash players at the English Institute of Sport in Sheffield. Lara, 28, has been with the team since November 2013 backing up Ross' work as head coach by providing information, background and analysis into player well-being, as well as personal and emotional development.

When it was time to go into the nets, which was when the playing squad were having their lunch, I took a stint facing up to Ross' underarm bowling with three pairs of goggles.

With the first pair of goggles (with the clearest vision), and although I'm pretty useless, I played one wonderful off drive through the covers and held the pose. The second pair (with reduced vision) I found to be the hardest to judge of the three and I made little impact as I found myself struggling. This was despite Ross giving me forewarning that he was delivering the ball. The third and final "blackout" goggles were a revelation as I found my hearing to be far more alert and profound. I had to listen carefully for the bearings in the ball in order to try and hit it.

All in all, I found my time with the team behind the England Visually Impaired Squad to be a pleasure; nothing proved too much hassle. A big thank you to all involved for a great day!

5. Wheelchair Rugby League

Despite being Welsh born and bred, I have never particularly been a fan of the oval ball game, especially Union. In fact, when I was working at Manchester United Television for eleven-and-a-half years, it was a common facet of office craic that someone would say I should really like the oval ball sport. My usual, rather stern riposte to this, was to rattle off a statistic that they were four times as many football clubs in the principality than rugby union clubs.

To further this point, I statistically found out that there are more cricket clubs in North Wales than Rugby Union by 39 to 32. I have always found it rather misleading and a common misconception by people hailing from all corners of the U.K. (and of the media) why football, (until Wales' stellar performance at Euro 2016, at least) has never been deemed the national sport. It clearly is, in my opinion, apart from a few weekends in January and February every year during the Six Nations, plus a few days every four years when Wales are playing in the rugby union World Cup.

Coming from the North East of Wales, so close to the footballing metropolises of Manchester and Liverpool, it is seldom that the round ball and the latest developments surrounding football aren't the main topics of discussion. Just like for the vast majority of England and Scotland.

Nonetheless, retaining a great fondness for the North West of England due to its geographical closeness, I have always maintained a great respect for the sport of rugby league and have always failed to fathom (a southern bias/divide aside) why rugby league isn't as widely followed in as many nations as its union counterpart.

The North Wales Crusaders Rugby League Wheelchair Team is based in Queensferry, Flintshire, and I got in touch with the then manager, Mark Jones, who is now the club's chairman. Mark has had a varied working career, to say the least. After being a firefighter in the North Wales Fire Service from 1978 to 2008, he gained a Fire Engineering Degree at, what is now known as, the University of Central Lancashire in 1995. After leaving the fire service, Mark changed careers by becoming a support worker before retraining as a maths teacher at Liverpool Hope University in 2011. After achieving his PGCE, Mark was a schoolteacher from June 2011 to November 2013 before going into freelance cycling coaching, within which he had worked concurrently with teaching from May 2012.

As manager of NWCWRL (North Wales Crusaders Wheelchair Rugby League), Mark secured promotion from the Western Division of the wheelchair league in his first season before consolidating with a third place out of four finish in the Premier League in 2016 behind Halifax and Leeds Rhinos. They travel as far afield as Medway, who finished fourth and bottom in 2016, in Kent.

However, the club for the 2018 season play in the Championship division along with teams from Manchester, Merseyside, Leyland in Lancashire, and Glasgow.

For the start of the 2018 season, the club has broadened in scope to include wheelchair basketball with the support of North Wales Basketball. In addition to this, North Wales Crusaders Wheelchair Rugby League is a charitable organisation and has attained Blue Ribbon status from Disability Sport Wales.

I arrived for the club's first training session of the 2017 season on Friday 20th January 2017 at Deeside Leisure Centre at about 5.30 pm for a 6 pm start. Upon arrival, I met two of the wheelchair coaches before ordering a mocha from the café as I was early; I usually am whenever I go somewhere

Deeside Leisure Centre has been the base of Welsh rugby league since May 2012 when Flintshire County Council entered into a 25-year partnership with Wales National Rugby League. Prior to this, the base was at Queensway Leisure Centre in Wrexham, where whilst taking part in my own sport of interval training, I shared the track with the Welsh national team during the autumn 2011 internationals against Australia, England and New Zealand.

The aim of the partnership is "to provide an elite training facility for the national squads supporting the development of North Wales age group teams."

Prior to my arrival at the training session, after researching online and discussing matters over the phone and email with Mark Jones, I knew I would take part in the session in a wheelchair. For you see, wheelchair rugby league is said to all-inclusive as it offers the disabled and non-disabled, across both sexes, the opportunity to compete with and against one another.

Wheelchair rugby league is usually played in a sports centre, taking up most of the length of the hall, and there are five players on each team. A completed pass over the try line, which is set out with cones, is classed as a score and conversions are made by punching the ball over mini rugby league posts from a tee. Tackles are made, as in tag rugby league, by bagging an attached tag or flag.

The running of North Wales Crusaders Wheelchair Rugby League is a community programme funded directly by the club's wheelchair and disability sports association. Every aspect of the club is taken care of by volunteers; from coaching, to administration, to press coverage and social media posting.

The club was formed in April 2013 to cater for those with disabilities following the enormous success of the Paralympics on home soil in London in 2012. There are two teams within the club. Firstly, a junior team from ages seven to 12. Then a senior team. In addition to this, eight of the club's senior squad were a part of Wales' triumphant Celtic Cup success in autumn 2016, including the Welsh captain, Mark Williams. More on Mark later. The wheelchairs the club use are designed especially for sport, and for young and old.

With all this in mind, I nervously entered the sports hall with the folder containing all my research to be given a coaching session, to test out my new wheels, by 40-year-old Claire Cranston. Claire, who isn't physically disabled, first got involved with the club after her friend asked her to attend an open day of the NWCWRL. Claire was a member of the side that won promotion from the Western Division in 2015. So far, she has scored six tries for the team and told me she finds playing the sport to be an excitement and a thrill. She enjoys the social aspect and the exercise that wheelchair rugby offers. Before Claire's friend insisted she attend the open day, Claire had never heard of the club.

As Claire was instructing me how to use the wheelchair, I found my initial movements to be slightly disconcerting as it played a little with my usual senses of space, perception, and movement that, as an able-bodied person, I shamefully take for granted. Walking and running in the traditional sense is a privilege. I should really know this with the physical difficulties my Ma has had in recent years.

The team session started with warm-up movements on the chair with instructions. One was forward, two backwards, and three sideways. In my initiation from Claire, I had found the latter movement by far the hardest. Following the group warm-up, we undertook shuttles or "suicides." Needless to state, despite my enthusiasm, I was the slowest by far!

Nonetheless, I was doing much better than I thought I would. However, I found spatial awareness quite a test. The camaraderie displayed amongst the group was fantastic as, despite my lack of wheelchair ability, I was greatly encouraged by each member of the group.

One in particular, who took time during the session to help and make me feel welcome was Stuart Williams, who hails from Wallasey on the

Wirral, but is the Welsh Wheelchair Rugby League vice-captain. I found Stuart to the biggest, most outgoing character in the team, but undoubtedly very obliging. Stuart scored 32 points during the 2016 season for NWCWRL in eight appearances, including two friendlies, playing from centre.

The encouragement I received from all the group, not just Stuart, even when I was in a collision with the captain of the Crusaders and Wales Wheelchair Rugby League, Mark Williams, was amazing. I was rather worried when Mark, who is a double amputee, fell out of his chair. At this point, I felt rather embarrassed, but Mark got back into his chair with a minimum of fuss that perhaps highly paid able-bodied athletes should take note of.

Mark is an extremely talented, heroic and polymathic man. He holds separate law and business/computer studies degrees from the University of Wales, Bangor. Currently, he is studying part-time for a Ph.D. from Nottingham Trent University in philosophy, military and operational law.

In addition to wheelchair rugby league, which included captaining Wales in the World Cup in 2017, he plays wheelchair rugby union for Wales, completed The BUPA Great North Run three times (2008, 2010 & 2012), and (possibly the most impressive of his sporting accomplishments) finished in the top six of Britain's Strongest Adaptive Man in 2015 and 2016. Last, but not least, Mark skydived 13,500 feet in August 2007 raising £1,500 for charity. In his working life, Mark has plied his trade for several multi-national companies.

I think you'll agree, judging by his many varied accomplishments, Mark Williams is a truly inspirational man. Mark's story and all the Crusaders wheelchair team show that there are no limits to life and the challenges you can overcome. They put most people to shame… able-bodied or otherwise.

After a tag game of wheelchair rugby league, where I was slightly disappointed, but not surprised, not to con my way to scoring a try, I left my chair to talk to three members of the junior team.

Firstly, I spoke to 12-year-old Mason, who is physically disabled and has cerebral palsy. Mason made his debut for the senior team during the 2016 season, but before joining the club, he told me of his lack of confidence. Mason's involvement with wheelchair rugby league helps take his mind off his difficulties whilst giving him a fun place to go and is a big highlight of his week, along with playing darts. Following Mason, I spoke to 13-year-old Scarlett, who also has cerebral palsy. She enjoys the social aspect and competition of wheelchair rugby league.

Finally, I spoke to 12-year-old Georgina, who has cerebral palsy and diplegia. Georgina found out about NWCWRL when the club was collecting money on the street to raise funds. She enjoys the physical aspect of wheelchair rugby league when "bashing" into opposition players. Whilst doing this, Georgina puts her energy into the session and pretends she is colliding with people that have been mean to her whilst going fast. This helps greatly after a bad day. The social aspect makes Georgina "feel like everyone else." In addition to wheelchair rugby league, Georgina plays wheelchair rugby union, which she had been doing during the close season.

These three young children undoubtedly prove to me what a fully inclusive club the NWCWRL is.

I said my goodbyes to everyone rather impressed at the level of skill, movement, and inclusivity displayed by members of the club. To famously quote The Smiths "…the pleasure, the privilege was mine" in meeting these people.

6. Wheely Good Fitness

In July 2017, six months after my visit to North Wales Crusaders Wheelchair Rugby League, and my attempts at getting to grips with being in a wheelchair (the eye-opening experience that was), I met Kris Saunders-Stowe of Wheely Good Fitness in a Starbucks on a 30C degree day in Ross-on-Wye in Herefordshire, where Kris is based.

Wheely Good Fitness is his company where he works as a fitness instructor. His unique selling point is that he focuses on clients with disabilities, some of whom face great barriers to taking part in exercise. Kris runs classes throughout Herefordshire for his clientele and also has personal training clients whom he has helped to complete long-distance endurance events, amongst other achievements.

I was driven and accompanied for the two-and-a-half hour car journey to see Kris by my mate, and former Ross on-Wye resident, Andrew Atkinson. In fact, it was Andrew who brought Kris to my attention when I was researching this book. He knew Kris from his time in Ross whilst being a councillor in the town.

I was not as prepared for meeting Kris as I normally would be. In fact, Andrew arrived at my home for our journey with me upstairs getting ready. This is very unlike me and I was even frantically writing questions down in the few minutes before Kris arrived.

In the fantastically warm British summer weather that we experience all too rarely (although it makes you feel alive, happy and proud to be British), I greeted Kris outside the Starbucks as I drank a mocha cooler, my favourite summer drink.

Despite being ill-prepared, by my standards, I did read one online interview where I was intrigued by some of Kris's tips on exercise. In fact, I found myself agreeing with him a lot. One segment of the interview that interested me was how Kris likes to have a one-to-one talk with clients before a class. Kris told me that he doesn't assume what adaptions have to be made for clients, many of whom have physical and emotional disabilities, including autism; they can range from instructions being delivered in a different way to helping clients alter equipment. He sees someone quite simply as an individual. He likes to focus on what someone can achieve rather than what they cannot.

Elaborating further, Kris's words resonated with me when he explained that independent is what you want to be. For some clients, lifting a coffee mug is a great step in their independence. This especially reverberated with me as many of the services that my family has encountered are intent on a 'one size fits all' approach, often because of budgetary constraints.

If needs be, Kris can introduce clients very slowly to his classes and exercise. This means they can just turn up the first time, and there is no need to actually take part. The first class can be a big stress for someone with a disability and is a feeling I've had many times in the past. This is due to the worry as to what lies ahead in the new environment. When the client eventually joins the class, they may be encouraged further by joining the cooldown to start with, or by having another few visits to the gym, or even just meeting Kris for a coffee.

When Kris was explaining all this, my life's experiences with training and exercise came vividly flooding back from my teenage years to the very recent past. When I was younger, I would have been glad to have Kris as an instructor that was so understanding.

Kris can also see that his classes become part of his clients' social lives and their routines. After a while, he sees their confidence improve. It's about the improvement in the long term for Kris; little improvements eventually become more noticeable and thus larger.

Kris started his company Wheely Good Fitness in 2013, as he felt that disability could be better promoted for people that weren't Paralympians. This was a change in career for him after spending his entire working life, from the age of 18, in retail. Kris uses a wheelchair himself and the name of the business was thought up by Kris's partner. Kris's condition is degenerative and affects his ability to walk unaided, although he isn't paralysed.

Although he has been advised to limit his exercise routine (he is only supposed to take part in one yoga session a week), he has taken on various gruelling physical challenges including twice using his wheelchair to go around the full 26.2 miles of the London Marathon course. In fact, Kris feels and believes that exercise can help his fatigue and pain management.

Kris's times were four hours, 54 minutes on the first occasion, and four hours, 24 minutes the second time around (even though he was suffering from a shoulder injury which severely curtailed his training). Kris's other achievements include skydiving, bungee jumping, zip wiring, and water sports, whilst there is a video online of Kris climbing a wall using an adapted wheelchair harness. In fact, Kris was part of a Channel Four series shown to coincide with the Rio 2016 Paralympics. He was even in a promo for the channel's coverage of the Paralympics appearing as a ballroom dancer.

Kris has also been invited, like myself, to Buckingham Palace as he won the Herefordshire Community Champion Award in 2016. He felt this to be a great honour as, in his childhood, his parents would insist that he stand for the national anthem whenever it was played on radio or television. He was also invited to 10 Downing Street for a reception held by Samantha Cameron as part of his work with the charity Scope.

Despite all Kris's daredevil stunts, accolades, and gruelling physical accomplishments, he tells me he is in pain "24/7" but the adaptability of having his own business enables him to undertake the hours he can physically do.

Meeting Kris was engaging, interesting and inspiring. Kris taught me that there are literally thousands of people who are inspirational in the United Kingdom, who have overcome great barriers, and who achieve many fantastic feats.

However, alongside Kris' great achievements and feats, it is his engaging, charming, helpful, and likeable personality that sets him aside from most. During the research for this book, and working on my autistic memoir, I have found or come across literally dozens of interesting and inspirational stories online (some of whom I contacted without getting anywhere, or in the flesh). However, it is his personality that makes Kris stand out ahead of many others I have encountered.

7. Autism and Exercise

As someone with autism, who is keen on exercise and its positive effects, I have often wondered about the amount and level of exercise that fellow autistic people experience.

To reach an elite level at any sport (or the levels required to be an incredible musician), you must often display traits of obsessive-compulsive disorder, autism, or a related condition. One of the world's best footballers – Lionel Messi – is alleged to have an autistic spectrum disorder and there have been unconfirmed stories regarding Grand Slam tennis champion, Rafael Nadal, having autism or traits thereof.

Nonetheless, for this book, I am more interested in so-called "regular" people with disabilities, and, for the purposes of this chapter, autism. In my rather small sample size, and the anecdotal evidence I have encountered regarding autistic people and exercise, it has often seemed that I am a bit of a lone ranger when it comes to autism and regular exercise. So, willing to prove my experiences to be an aberration, or not the correct or full picture, I contacted Amy Webster from Active for Autism to find out about her experiences in her role working with people with autism who like and attend regular exercise training sessions.

Amy's role at The National Autistic Society, which is based in Leeds, is to coordinate the Active for Autism project. This involves developing and delivering autism training courses specifically for sport and physical activity leaders (coaches, PE teachers, volunteers, etc.), with the aim of increasing the number of autism spectrum people playing sport.

According to Amy, there isn't really such a thing as a 'typical work day' in her job. Nonetheless, the main part of her job is to be out delivering the training to sport and activity leaders. Amy's work can head down a variety of formats, so she can either be out delivering for two days, one day, or half a day, depending on what is requested. She often commences any session by giving an overview of autism before going on to discuss how autism can affect participation in sport and physical activity. On the majority of courses, Amy will also lead some physical activities to allow course participants to work through some suggested strategies and adaptations that can be used to train someone with autism.

Should Amy find herself 'in the office' rather than out delivering, then she will either be attending meetings, looking at ways to further develop training, or working on additional materials. For example, The NAS is producing a 'good practice' resource to accompany the training.

One really nice success story is of a player at Danby Rovers; it has stuck in Amy's mind. The player struggled with social interaction and didn't feel confident in a big group or team environment. But, following a team trip to London, Amy saw a huge increase in the player's confidence and they have since attended more social outings with the team (bowling, meals, etc.), as well as going on to join additional social clubs besides football.

Amy explained that the benefits of exercise are well known – it can help people increase self-esteem, develop social skills, and improve physical and mental health, as well as general wellbeing. It is also important to consider the additional benefits that exercise may have on people with certain disabilities or differences such as:

- Improved stamina and muscle strength to improve balance and coordination

- The endorphins released during exercise can offer a natural 'feel good' high which may help to reduce anxiety or combat depression

- Participating in group activities, or even individual sports in a group environment, can be a way to promote social interaction and make new friends

- Participating in sport or physical activity can provide people with a great deal of independence.

Amy has also encountered individuals who have witnessed a number of psychological benefits from exercise and sport such as an improvement of mood, a reduction in anxiety and depression, and an increase in self-esteem. She has worked with autistic people who, in the past, haven't had any social interaction with others or who haven't had the confidence to try new activities. However, when approached in the right way (such as coaches introducing new activities in familiar environments) then physical activity can be a great starting point for trying new experiences.

In addition to her role with Active for Autism, Amy is a volunteer football coach with the Leeds-based pan-disability football club, Danby Rovers. She works in a voluntary capacity as secretary and coach of the club.

Her responsibilities include coaching for four hours per week as well as providing opportunities for competitive football for those people who wish to play against other teams. Aside from the football coaching responsibilities, Amy also works with the other volunteers to provide additional sessions for the players covering topics such as money management, personal hygiene, healthy eating, drugs and alcohol, respect, using public transport, and more. She is a very busy lady!

One player to have gained from training and playing for Danby Rovers is 23-year-old James McKenna. James got into football through college back in 2009 and has played for eight years. He found out about Danby Rovers DFC through his tutors at college, as one of them is a coach at the club.

When it comes to being in a group – which many autistic people can find overpowering and very difficult – James, however, loves this aspect. In fact, he goes on to say that he "loves every second of it." Moreover, James has learnt new skills, improved his fitness, and he has "made a lot of friends along the way in the eight years that I have played." Sport and exercise have helped James not only to get fitter, but it has also given him "confidence in life – to look for work" which is a burning political issue with autistic people at the moment. Indeed, James' newfound confidence enabled him to secure a job in a 1,000 student school as a cleaner.

Like I explained earlier in the book, James' experiences are similar to what I encountered in my time following Welsh Premier club, Cefn Druids. The players – who I was allowed to train with twice every week even though I was 'only' a supporter – treated me with great respect and understanding, and for the first time in my life up until that juncture, I felt appreciated, cared about, and respected outside my close family.

As someone who struggles when illness, inclement weather, or any event that can affect training occurs, I was intrigued to know if these kinds of things affect James. He told me that he can be "disappointed [when not training] but work has to come first because I get paid to work and I don't get paid to play football." With regard to inclement weather, "When a scheduled round of matches at Preston got cancelled last weekend due to the weather… it did affect me a little bit but I made up for it in training the next day, putting in extra effect."

James told me that he has made, "lots of friends over the last eight years or so from training. We go out for drinks, and we go to the cinema and bowling."

For coaches, teachers, and activity leaders interested in learning more about the NAS's sport and physical activity programmes, further information is available at www.autism.org.uk/active

Another autism organisation that helps clients on the road to a fit and healthy lifestyle is Sheffield-based Autism Plus. Their fitness programmes are run in association with local leisure organisation Access Fitness, which claims to be the UK's first specialist disability and mental health-focused gym. The gym itself is located at the Wellness Centre at the Concord Sports Centre in Sheffield.

Access Fitness also runs, in partnership with the Sheffield United Community Foundation and SIV, the Concord Sports Centre. Amongst the facilities offered is a structured training programme, led by qualified personal trainers with a background in disability and mental health support. A one-to-one session with a trainer costs £23 for an hour's workout.

Access Fitness's work specifically caters for the needs of individuals with disabilities and mental health diagnoses so they "can exercise in a more comfortable, welcoming environment." The gym space is designed to be centred around the individual person's needs, is user-friendly, and easy to navigate with colour-coded footprints. The equipment is also adapted to suit the user's requirements as part of the gym experience.

Individual exercise plans are drawn up that are "fun and personal" helping the autistic person, or individual with mental health difficulties, to access a healthier lifestyle. Members also have the option of either one-to-one support or small exercise groups. Family members are also welcome to attend sessions.

In addition to the link up with Access Fitness, Autism Plus runs a Community Health Champions Programme where volunteers are given a role to support people to eat healthily, be physically active, and improve their mental wellbeing. The Community Health Champions Programme project is supported by several voluntary and community organisations, Sheffield City Council, and the local NHS. Each Champion gets training, support, and valuable work experience. Champions must be able to commit to volunteering for 16 hours a month for at least six months, as well as attending some training. The project is designed to help people to live healthier lives by providing activities, information, and support, and to help make the community in Sheffield a healthier place.

All in all, it is nice to know that there are such excellent facilities and programmes offered specifically for people with autism. In my opinion, this is further fuel to my belief that the general public's awareness is at an all-time high. As far as exercise is concerned, these are big steps in the right direction. In the future, there should be more help and support to encourage people with autism to live healthier lifestyles. A 2016 research study from the U.K. charity, Autistica, stated that even "high-functioning" autistic people can die up to 18 years earlier than the average life expectancy.

Surely, exercise for the higher functioning on the spectrum, and a healthier lifestyle, will add to their life expectancy whilst helping those who have depression and anxiety issues, which I believe go hand in hand with the condition.

Schemes such as those discussed in this chapter should, in my opinion, become more commonplace in the future. Although it will cost money initially, it is my undoubted belief that the schemes will save money in the long run, reduce dependency on the National Health Service, and lengthen lives for those with autism.

8. Cwm Wanderers F.C. Autism Academy

Whilst looking for more information on autistic people taking part in sport, and finding the research harder than expected (I found myself turned down for contributions or initial contact emails amounted to nothing), I was delighted to receive an email from Andrea Smith in October 2017. Andrea helps run a football club called Cwmtwrch Wanderers, or Cwm Wanderers as they are more commonly referred to. Andrea has been involved with the club for six years, and her husband Kevin is the club secretary; they started the mini and junior sections of the club with their youngest son, Jac, when he was 4. Andrea has been involved ever since, and the mini and junior sections have flourished.

The club itself was formed in 1931 upon the establishment of the Neath Football League. They relocated to their new ground, at Parc Afon Twrch, in summer 2013 as their previous base in Brynderi was part of a project to build a primary school.

I had got in touch with the club after reading an article regarding the fascinating academy they had formed during the summer of 2017. This wasn't just your regular academy (Cwm already has seven junior teams ranging from age six to 18, and a reserve team that acts as a feeder for their record 16-time Neath League title-winning first team) but more interestingly an autism academy in conjunction with the Swansea City F.C. Community Trust.

First of all, I asked 41-year-old Andrea how the idea of the academy came about. She explained, "My son Steffan is 16 and has autism. A year ago, Steffan asked me if he could join our local football team. As much as I was delighted that he was taking an interest in something, I knew that he wouldn't cope with being shouted at from the sideline, taking on-board multiple instructions at once and fitting in.

"To be honest, I just made excuses as to why he couldn't join. Autism isn't a condition that's widely understood, and so I knew, in my heart, that it would be a disaster. I really wanted to do something to help him get involved in a community-based sporting activity. So, I thought, what if we could create a development academy to sit alongside a mainstream team to coach on a smaller scale with a specialist coach that would develop Steffan's skills, and give him the experience he needs to enjoy being in a mainstream team?

"My idea was what if we then trained the mainstream coach to be autism aware, and ease the move across from the academy to the mainstream?

What if we trained the whole squad to be autism aware and help Steffan fit in? How amazing and life-changing could that be for not only my son, but every child with autism who joined the academy, as well as their families? Cwm Wanderers jumped at the chance to be involved in such a life-changing project. The club chairman Kerry Williams, vice-chairman Derrick Britain, and treasurer Stewart Evans have just been so supportive. This is in addition to the main committee and women's committee at the club. They cannot do enough to support this project, and we are very lucky to have them all on-board.

"So, in March 2017, an opportunity presented itself to myself and my work colleague, Louise, at our business. We are both operations managers at EE, who are owned by BT, in Merthyr Tydfil. The competition was in the form of a BT Dragon's Den. It was just like the Dragon's Den on TV where you pitch an idea to get the backing of the Dragons and, if they like it, they help you implement it. The brief for the competition was to bring technology and sport together to improve the lives of disadvantaged people. I thought to myself, now this is a great competition and would be a perfect vehicle to allow me to progress the idea of the academy. I talked it over with Louise. She had already met Steffan, as he had previously been to EE on work experience, and so she understood his limitations. She thought it was an excellent idea and one that she was so passionate to help with.

"After meeting and working with Steffan, Louise became aware of how hard it is for him to communicate and she really wanted to help him with this. We pitched our proposal to the Dragons, presenting our idea to set up an academy for children like Steffan which would mirror a mainstream football team, but which would be exclusively for children and young people on the ASD spectrum. They would go to weekly training sessions run by specialist coaches, followed by a range of social activities in the clubhouse. They would be able to buy snacks, listen to music, and make friends without feeling ridiculed or picked on, which is the greatest barrier for them. We wanted to create an app especially for these children to help keep them engaged, track their fitness, and record their training success by awarding club points for them to redeem against drinks and snacks. Our ambition was for the Academy to give young people like Steffan a chance to learn skills on and off the field; the ultimate goal would be for them to successfully secure their place in a mainstream team.

"After the pitch, a visitor approached us from the Swansea City Community Trust Football Club. He was in the audience supporting another pitch. He was so impressed with our project that he asked me if we would consider a partnership with the Swans and they would help us bring our project to life. He really felt that this project was amazing. We didn't hesitate to say yes! And that's exactly what we have done. We have set up the first development academy of this kind exclusively for children with ASD in Wales. We have been working extremely hard since March this year to secure specialist coaches through Disability Sports Wales, engaging my local football club – Cwm Wanderers ACF – who agreed to be the first club to trial it. We created a brand to reflect our ambition and we reached out to the local community to gauge interest in the project. We were overwhelmed with the number of children who wanted to sign up and we opened the academy on Saturday the 2nd of September at a huge event at the club. More than 500 people attended the event, and it was a massive success. We haven't quite finished everything yet. BT and EE are in the process of installing broadband into the club so that the children will be able to use their iPads at the club to utilise the app. We have also set up a project team combining the skills of staff at EE and BT working collaboratively to develop this. This is the next phase of the project, and we hope the app will be ready by the end of January 2018. That will complete the initial set up of the very first academy of its kind, focusing specifically on inclusion rather than separation. The response from families in our community who are affected by ASD has convinced us that this is exactly the sort of project that is needed."

Training sessions began in September 2017, with 20 places set aside for the 2017-18 season, and plans to extend the scheme to 40 participants in Year Two enabling what Andrea believed would be, "a realistic level to begin with, as this is a new project."

Furthermore, the very different needs of autistic people are of paramount importance to Andrea as she explains that, "It's extremely important to us that we get to know each child individually before we take a new one on, so that we understand each child's needs. Each volunteer has been trained at the club and we personally get to know each and every child before a new one joins.

"We currently have 17 children attending the academy with a waiting list to fill it. It will be full by the end of January 2018. It was always our intention to ramp up slowly to ensure its success. Most of the children are local with three children traveling 15 miles to attend."

As someone who worked for the television channel of Manchester United for just over 11 years and, while personally having good experiences, especially in my younger years, I wondered how helpful Swansea City F.C. had been in assisting Cwm Wanderers and Andrea in the start-up of the academy.

"We have had support both directly from Swansea City FC in addition to the Swansea City Community Trust. The trust are part of the BT Supporters Club but work alongside Swansea City FC. The trust have provided funding to us for the first year to start the academy; Swansea City FC Academy Manager Nigel Rees has also supported us by providing us with training kits, playing kits, and equipment to help us start. Nigel brought some academy players to the event on the launch day to meet the children and show a Swans presence at launch day. They also presented the children with signed footballs too, which the children loved. The Trust also supported us on launch day and sent representation to us to referee football games. They have also provided us with match tickets for our children and are in touch with us regularly to offer support. Both the trust and the Swans Academy have been fantastic."

I asked Andrea how the autistic players have mixed with one another. By way of context, I can be very competitive with autistic people of a similar age, although I am not like this with the small children I volunteer with at a Wrexham-based autism charity called Your Space (I have to be the responsible one!).

"In the main, they cope really well. We have one coach who is specially trained in disability, but alongside that, we have two of my other sons helping out volunteering, as well as two of their friends. So we have four children who are not autistic, working with the group. My middle son, Rhys, is 15 and volunteers both for the football training and in the youth club. He is already autism-aware while being trained with specific football skills from my husband Kevin, who is Cwm Wanderer's club secretary and an established coach, so that he can bring these coaching skills across to the session.

"My youngest son, Jac, is ten. He also volunteers at football and attends youth club with two of his friends. These three children have been in the same football team since they were five in Cwm Wanderer's mainstream team. The coach utilises them during the session to demonstrate specific skills learning and one-on-one training for the children. This works really well as we have children from the mainstream teams interacting with the academy to raise awareness of autism so that the academy children can feel at home at any time in the club.

"There is some competition both in the team and during youth club and sometimes this can cause some tension, but our volunteers have got to know each child and can identify issues before they begin. We then use coping strategies to help calm down any situation which may arise. In the main, the football session is controlled very well with very little disruption as everyone plays their part in ensuring the session runs smoothly."

I was intrigued by the youth club idea, for the reasons I've explained above, and asked Andrea if she could elaborate on the youth club that takes place after a training session.

"The youth club is an activity-based club to help encourage communication, interaction, and create a fun environment that the children can attend directly after training. We offer activities such as pool, Wii Games, arts and crafts, board games, and the like, to encourage participation. After the football, all children attend the youth club where we have a discussion about a topic of our choice to encourage conversation and then the children are rewarded for taking part in this. Then we have a feelings board so that each child can put an emoji on it to describe how they are feeling. We also have a song board that they all put one song a week on, for our own playlist, which plays in the background.

"After the discussion, all the children break off to participate in the activities we offer. For the older children, we offer assistance to help set them up for work. We let them stand behind the bar with us and serve the children pop, crisps, and chocolate so that it develops their customer-facing skills, as well as handling money, which we feel would be beneficial to them once they leave school. We show them how to use a till and how to interact with customers."

As well as the training sessions, I asked Andrea if there were any plans for the autistic youngsters to play matches against opposing clubs in either friendlies or a league.

"We are planning a Disability through Sport Awareness Day in April 2018 which will incorporate a fun day of football, games, and a music festival while our academy will play a disability team within our area. That is in its early stages of planning at the moment. The whole purpose of the academy is to upskill the children in preparation for the mainstream, then coach the mainstream coach on how to instruct the child, and then integrate them over to the mainstream so that we are an inclusive club. Some children in our academy may never make that leap, but we will be organising games next season for them."

Personally, when I was a young child (I am now 33) there was nothing of this ilk to encourage me to be a part of; few knew of autism in the 1990s. I'd like to think it may have been an escape, for me, from the disrupted schooling I had.

We are currently in an era of significant cuts to services in the public sector for people with disabilities, including autism. In addition, 70% of autistic schoolchildren are in mainstream schools, and many struggle in these environments. Often, staff are not fully equipped to deal with their additional needs. Nonetheless, it is hugely comforting to know that the autistic youngsters in Cwmtwrch have Cwm Wanderers F.C. Autism Academy to play for in their social time, due to the great thinking and ingenuity of Andrea Smith.

9. Wrexham Boxing Club

For many generations, the sport of boxing has been renowned for instilling a sense of discipline into many of its exponents. Many boxers may otherwise have gone down the wrong path in life; boxing helps provide a way to get their angst and frustrations out in a controlled environment.

Although many professional boxers have suffered well-publicised problems after retirement when the structure of organised intensive training has ended, it begs the question as to how these people would have coped without the competitive nature of sport giving them somewhere to go, and a reason to get up, each morning in their younger years.

With all this clearly in my mind, I remembered a gentleman named George Crewe, who worked at St. Christopher's Special School in my youth and who had coached Joe Calzaghe in his Welsh international amateur boxing days. As a youngster with behavioural problems at the time (due to my autism), and bad experiences at the schools I attended, I really respected George. George had a great rapport and understanding with many pupils at the school, who came from extremely troubled backgrounds; backgrounds that were far more troubled than mine ever was.

In fact, over the years, George has attracted some of the pupils he has worked with at St. Christopher's to the boxing club which has helped them enormously with their mental health, as well as their additional learning needs. In fact, one of the other coaches at the club is also currently a teaching assistant at St. Christopher's, thus keeping a link between the club and the school.

Although slight of stature with white hair and, at this time, in his mid-sixties, George maintained a presence that endeared him greatly to the pupils. He would take part in gardening sessions at the school and seemed fit as a fiddle – belying his age. I knew at this stage, at the turn of the millennium, that George was still active at Wrexham Boxing Club. Long after I left St. Christopher's, he would greet my Ma and sister Mel, who worked with me at the school, at the local supermarket in a very friendly way.

So, fondly remembering George and with this book developing in early 2017, Mel suggested that I see if George was still with the club. I knew he was still involved with St. Christopher's (gardening with the pupils on a Friday) and that he was now approaching his octogenarian years. I found an email and phone number for the club that I assumed was George's.

After a couple of conversations to arrange a time to go down to the club, I met up with George on Monday 20th February 2017.

When I entered the club, I saw the walls were adorned with pictures of club trainers with Welsh former World Cruiserweight Champion Enzo Maccarinelli and, of course, obligatory pictures of the recently-departed Muhammad Ali (including the famous shot of the Sonny Liston fight on 25th February 1964). At this point, I greeted George who recognised my brother-in-law Bill and my Ma, but failed to recognise me fully; I have lost weight, and grown both facial and hair "up top" since leaving St. Christopher's in July 2003. Upon eventually recognising me, George regaled me with a story of how I used to come out of my classroom quite sternly, but that he always knew how to say a calming word to me. We also talked about the other characters we encountered at the school and how their lives developed in the ensuing years.

George has been involved with Wrexham Boxing Club since its inception in 1982. He found the area lacked a boxing club when he left the Royal Air Force in around 1959, so he eventually decided – 23 years later – to form his own club. In its 35-year history, the club has led a rather peripatetic existence around the town; it was first at Wrexham Victoria, then Wrexham Swimming Baths (now Waterworld) in a room below the diving board, the former Flex Gym (which I used to frequent as a child), Wrexham Industrial Estate, Sports Connect and on the former site of The Groves school.

At its height, the club had around 70 members, but now has "around 50," although there were slightly fewer on the night I was there "due to the school holidays." When I asked George how many have passed through the various doors of the club since 1982, he said that he had seen "literally thousands."

A slight adjunct to Wrexham Boxing Club's history is that during the build-up to London 2012, Wrexham played host to the Lesotho Olympic squad who trained at Wrexham Boxing Club. Furthermore, all Lesotho's athletes trained in the town in preparation for the 2014 Commonwealth Games in Glasgow. On the former occasion, I personally bumped into 200-metre runner Mesito Lehata at Queensway track whilst I was running. Lehata's impressive claim to fame is beating Usain Bolt in the heats of the 2013 World Championships in Moscow. However, after grabbing the ultimate scalp, Lehata was eliminated in the semi-finals.

Unfortunately, in 2013, with the old school set for demolition, which as of late 2016 is now a listed building, Wrexham Boxing Club was without a home again. In May 2013, when it looked like they might have to close their doors for the final time, Steve Williams, youth coach at the club, made an appeal in the local press:

"We don't need anything pretty [regarding a new venue]. If we can source a secure, affordable, weatherproof building with enough space to hold a ring and our bag equipment, we can use our limited funds - and maybe tap into a grant scheme - to make the improvements needed. We just really need a shell. But if we don't find anywhere in a few weeks, it could be the end for us."

So, with this in mind, Wrexham County Borough Council took the club "under its wing." Initially, they suggested the club use nearby Rhosddu Community Centre, but members of the club deemed it unsuitable due to various factors including lack of space, cost, and limited availability. In addition to this, Rhosddu Community Centre only had space for a 15-foot ring and four punch bags with numbers limited "to about a dozen." Also, the venue was only for hire for two sessions a week with the subs not enough to cover room hire.

With the club's future an issue on the agenda of a confidential meeting of Wrexham County Borough Council in June 2013, which the public and press were prohibited from attending, it was decided that Nice Acre Field Pavilion was to be the club's new home.

At this stage, it was hoped that it would take "six to eight weeks" following final council approval for the club to move to Nine Acre Fields, however, up until February 2014, the lease hadn't been signed which meant that Wrexham ABA had missed a season of action resulting in boxers training at various venues in Wrexham. Nonetheless, all was thankfully sorted and Wrexham Boxing Club had a new home.

The fact that the club is still running must be a blessed relief for its patrons, many of whom took time out to talk to me about their reasons for attending sessions.

The first person I talked to was Tom Pendlebury. Twenty-year-old Tom originates from Blackpool, but has been working on the building of HMP Berwyn on Wrexham Industrial Estate as an electrician. When it opened in February 2017, HMP Berwyn housed Category C adult male offenders and is said to be the joint biggest prison in the U.K. alongside HMP Oakwood in the Midlands.

Furthermore, when it comes to his boxing training, Tom likes the individual aspect of the sport and that, "the onus is down to you and, unlike team sports, no-one can let you down." He also enjoys the "in your face aspect of boxing," as he believes it to be a "school of hard knocks."

Following Tom, 22-year-old local resident Ben Ince, who is a builder by trade, took time out of his session to speak to me. Ben had been training for eight months in his second spell at Wrexham Boxing Club when I visited. Ben enjoys the discipline that it has instilled in him whilst "keeping him healthy." Nonetheless, after his first spell ended, and he stopped training at Wrexham Boxing Club, Ben freely admitted to me that he "lost discipline" as "he was out drinking with mates." Fortunately, he has now returned to the club and "takes out his aggression on the punchbags" in a positive, constructive manner rather than in a way that might not be so disciplined.

The third adult member of the club that I spoke to, gave me another insight into why he trains at the club. 28-year-old Richard Belton can't spar after being diagnosed with epilepsy. Although Richard hasn't had a fit in a decade, the risk is deemed too much by George and the other volunteer coaches to put him into the ring to spar or to fight.

Fortunately, though, Richard gets other positives from training at the club. Previously, he had played football for Brymbo, and after stopping playing he told me he "needed more exercise." He was advised to join the club by a mate of his and finds the time the club is held – on Monday and Wednesday evenings – suits his lifestyle as a support worker working nights with people with disabilities. Richard enjoys the "controlled aggression" of his boxing training and the competition with "a few of the lads keeping each other going."

After the three adults, I spoke to the youngsters from the club. However, they can only have three bouts in a year with fights lasting for just three one-minute rounds. The youngest age that someone can competitively box is ten in Wales and 11 in England. Currently, Wrexham Boxing Club has two Welsh national schoolboy champions and four Welsh internationals representing the club in various bouts and tournaments across the country.

Firstly, I chatted with 14-year-old Wrexham-based Aaron. He had been at the club for 18 months. Whilst I watched from the other end of the gym, I could see that, in my opinion, Aaron was the most technically talented and most developed of the youngsters who were present on the evening. Clearly, this was an opinion at least partly shared by the trainers at the club as he is one of four youngsters currently boxing for the club.

Aaron told me the reasons he boxes are "for self-defence and to keep me off the streets." He then elaborated further to use the word that was regularly offered to me during the evening for why people attended the club… "discipline." The discipline that clubs like this instil in people cannot and must not be underestimated. The help it offers youngsters and adults that may struggle to find the "right road" in life is fantastic and, in some people's cases, it must have changed their lives irrevocably.

In fact, Aaron himself went off the rails at one point and told me "he had fallen in with the wrong crowd" that saw him re-evaluate himself. The discipline from his boxing has seen Aaron excel at other sports, and he plays rugby union for Wrexham Youngsters and RGC East.

Finally, I chatted with 13-year-old Dylan, who has been training at the club "for five years on and off." Boxing offers Dylan an escape from school as he actually prefers attending the club to school. He then told me, with a twinkle in his eye, that he is only "sometimes" well behaved.

I am struck by how positive a community club like Wrexham Boxing Club can be for its local area. With Wrexham, the town I've lived in all my life, making such negative national headlines regarding long-term substance misuse in the town's bus station (as I write this in March 2017), I am saddened that places like Wrexham Boxing Club don't get the positive headlines they deserve. It doesn't make the news.

Also, as I write this, a "pioneering project" in the town will use football to tackle anti-social behaviour. The scheme has been funded by The Proceeds of Crime Act and The Office of the North Wales Police and Crime Commissioner. It will take place on Fridays between 7 and 9 pm, as that is when most anti-social behaviour takes place for 16- to 25-year-olds.

The sessions will be run by The Racecourse Community Foundation, which currently holds projects designed to increase physical activity, improve health and wellbeing, improve literacy and numeracy standards, and educate participants on diet, smoking, drugs and alcohol.

George Crewe has been doing something similar with boxing in the area for 35 years and has never won any awards. There are many of George's ilk around the U.K. helping youngsters stay out of trouble when successive governments short-sightedly cut public funding on projects that help the young have somewhere to go, gain discipline, and eventually respect their peers and elders.

People like George Crewe show dedication without recompense and help steer the development of youngsters and adults, who may otherwise have not had help. There are dozens of Georges, in different areas of society, who never get much praise. So, I want to say a big thank you to George, and the others like him, out there!

10. Joey Jones

When I was seven-years-old, it was arranged for me to answer questions on the history of Manchester United in The Black Horse Pub in our local village. The aim of this was to raise much-needed funds for my then school – Special Education Centre – in Wrexham. I correctly answered all 20 questions posed to me by the quizmaster, Liverpool FC European Cup Winner Joey Jones.

My answering of the questions was energetic – to say the least – and I still have a copy on DVD, converted from VHS, of the evening. The audience in the pub found it amusing, in an endearing manner, that a child so young had the ability to correctly answer questions of this ilk. I have, in recent times, given the footage of this to close mates as a present for birthdays and Christmases. In addition, a young Robbie Savage, who is from the same village as me, was present in the pub that evening.

On top of the 25 years I've personally know Joey, my Ma has known him and his wife Janice for well over four decades. So, with this in mind, and when I was scratching my head regarding dovetailing the exercise and illness angle of this book, Joey's name understandably came up. More regarding that later.

Joey's impressive playing career spanned 19 years with 594 Football League appearances for Wrexham (three spells), his childhood heroes, Liverpool, Chelsea and Huddersfield Town. Amongst his many successes were winning the League title and European Cup in 1977 with Liverpool and becoming, in the process, the first Welshman to win a winner's medal in Europe's Premier Competition. He also won 72 caps for his country, at the time being Wales' most capped player. The long-standing friend of our family had clearly been at the very top of his profession.

In addition to this, Joey has forged a long-standing friendship with ex-Manchester United (and many other clubs besides) winger Mickey Thomas. Their close bond has remained intact through their various adventures for over 45 years. They first bonded on a train journey from Colwyn Bay to Wrexham for their first day at the club, and have been inseparable ever since, whatever has been thrown their way in life.

Like Joey, over the years, Mickey has kept himself in great physical shape. I have an interesting anecdote that validates this. When I was at my desk in the M.U.T.V. office in early 2010, Mickey was there after filming a programme that morning at The Hilton Hotel near to our Deansgate base. I jokingly asked Mickey if he was still in decent physical condition. There and then, he took off his shirt to reveal his rather toned torso!

Back to Joey. We met on Friday the 12th of May 2017, just after 11 am, on a rather rainy morning, in the boardroom of Wrexham F.C.

In the club boardroom, I was immediately struck by a pennant from the European Cup Winners Cup Second Round, Second Leg tie, against my beloved Manchester United at The Racecourse on Wednesday 7th November 1990. This was the first season that English clubs were allowed back into European competition after a five year ban and, curiously enough, at this time, Wrexham were seeded higher in Europe than United. That season (1990-91), United won the Cup Winners Cup by beating Barcelona at the De Kuip Stadium in Rotterdam and Wrexham finished bottom of the Football League but were, fortunately, not relegated.

Also adorning the walls of Wrexham's boardroom were other pennants from their European adventures and photographs of the full internationals to have represented the club. Such an impressive collection rather belied their current status of being in the National League, the fifth tier of the English footballing pyramid, where they have been since 2008.

I came into the meeting wondering how exercise and sport had been the key to Joey's life. According to his 2005 memoir, Oh Joey, Joey! he had a rather eventful upbringing on a council estate in the seaside town of Llandudno; he was in a gang and occasionally ran into trouble with the authorities.

Joey told me that football was an outlet for him. It was a way to positively socialise and gain a life (be it on the streets) by having bags down as goalposts on the field near his estate, in the local five-a-side league, school matches, or by playing for Llandudno Estates in the Tremorfa League.

In addition to this, Joey engaged in his own exercise/sporting passion of boxing and sparred at Dyffryn ABA Club in Llandudno in his youth. He told me, "I most admire boxers and, apart from football, is the only other sport I take any interest in."

A story I heard off a player was about Joey once coaching at Wrexham. At a Royal Marine camp in Weymouth one pre-season, Joey was in the gym with a marine and kept up with his session. Subsequently, the marine suggested that he try one of Joey's sessions. He couldn't keep up with Joey!

In 2002, a heart condition manifested itself and required surgery. His surgeon informed Joey, "If you hadn't been so fit, you would have been dead." The surgeon also revealed that Joey would have unknowingly had this condition (to do with an aortic valve) during his illustrious playing days. Joey informed me that he had, "two aortic valves, rather than the usual three and I could have dropped dead at any moment." Medicals in his playing days, according to Joey, used to concern "only the hips down." Mickey's reaction to Joey's predicament, when he visited him in the hospital, was to characteristically joke and state that, "I didn't know you had a heart, Joe!"

Although Joey's rehabilitation was long, he told me, "It greatly helped my recovery that I had trained all my life." The working out afterwards, although to a lesser degree, and being involved with the lads at Wrexham, helped his recovery; he had missed the training and camaraderie that a football changing room undoubtedly provides. Joey loved the fact that this environment "was not sombre" and "love of the craic" further aided his progress.

When he went back to the gym with weight training in rehab, the weights were "the size of a pepper pot" according to Joey. He was unaccustomed to such small dumbbells. He also returned to punching the boxing bags. It is here that Joey credits a gentleman named Mal Purchase, who "spurred" him on after his illness.

Doctors told Joey, at the beginning of his recovery, that, "If you have to walk fifty yards, you have to remember to give enough energy for the return fifty yards." At this point, the determination that saw Joey succeed in his football career kicked in. "When you're told you can only run a mile, I'd run two, then four. That was the determination in me." He also freely admits that, "If I had been going into exercise for the first time after illness, and if I hadn't trained before, it would have been a shock to the system. Someone doing that would find it more difficult."

Although Joey has managed his heart condition over the last 15 years, he no longer trains due to another illness. Nonetheless, he told me how, "Training is addictive and now I've had to stop, I can see how people have to be weaned off it. Training releases stress and with it comes the endorphins. People should keep fit as it has helped me greatly and I wouldn't have changed my approach to training if I lived again."

On Wednesday 5th July 2017, Joey announced he was retiring from full-time coaching with Wrexham, but would continue on a part-time basis. He has given his life over to football, and he is entitled to be extremely proud of what he has achieved at the very elite end of the sport while helping many players break into Wrexham's first team over a quarter of a century. He deserves to enjoy taking this step back.

11. Charlotte Roach and Rabble

On a bright late winter's day, in a coffee shop next door to where I agreed to publish my memoirs with Bennion Kearny in the middle of Chester, I nervously waited for Charlotte Roach. With my autism, I always worry when I am waiting to meet anyone (even close friends that I have known over a decade) in case, at the last minute, they can't make it. I'm always at least 15 minutes early whenever I meet a mate or someone with work. It must stem from being born three weeks premature!

However, I needn't have worried. Charlotte arrived four minutes early for our meeting which, in my book, is a very impressive trait. I greeted Charlotte as she glanced around to see if I had already arrived. We make our introductions and go to the counter to order our coffees. I ask her about her time at Christleton High School in Chester between 2000 and 2007 and if she knew a teacher that worked there who is related to one of my best friends. Charlotte remembers the person I ask about, but is more vivid about their partner, who came along on a school trip. I've met him several times myself and he is quite a character.

Even before meeting Charlotte, and her being a great timekeeper, I was impressed after researching her story. Her tale is a very interesting one. Charlotte is a former Olympic triathlete hopeful who was mentored by Athens 2004 Olympic Double Gold medallist Dame Kelly Holmes as a youngster.

However, her London 2012 dream was ended with a near-fatal car accident, sustained whilst in a cycling session. At this point, Charlotte was training 30 hours a week with her "whole life" based around training. In fact, even as a child she trained between 13 and 14 hours at swimming alone, per week, which she freely admitted was "long and repetitive."

The near-fatal car accident saw a Land Rover travelling in the opposite direction hit Charlotte. She was in agony and struggling to breathe. A passing motorist stopped to help, and as luck would have it, it was Julie Hayton, a Leicester Tigers physiotherapist who was fortunately trained in CPR. Charlotte was gargling blood as Julie, realising there was a short window to help Charlotte, sat her up. This could have paralysed Charlotte, but it saved her life. However, Charlotte's injuries were very severe as both her lungs had collapsed, her back was broken in 12 places, and she'd suffered a broken collarbone. Charlotte spent a week in intensive care.

The great life-saving care Charlotte received from Derbyshire, Leicestershire & Rutland Air Ambulance after the accident prompted her to cycle solo 16,000 km from Beijing to London in August 2011 raising £9,000 for them. In addition to this, in 2016 Charlotte wore fancy dress every day for Lent to raise funds for London Air Ambulance.

At the time of her accident, Charlotte was in her second year studying at Cambridge University. She was running and swimming competitively and had been invited to join the UK Triathlon Programme for London 2012.

After the accident, Charlotte was frustrated at her inactivity, but miraculously returned to finish fourth in the European Cup Triathlon in 2010. Whilst participating in this event, Charlotte could feel the metalwork in her back jarring, but she wanted to prove to herself she could still race. However, training and competing ultimately became too much as she completed her neuroscience degree at Cambridge University.

From meeting Charlotte, I found it apparent that she knew, at least a little, of how to deal with autism from the way she conducted herself with me in a very understanding manner. At times, I can come across as quite overpowering, especially for people younger than me. The unperturbed manner with which Charlotte interacted with me might be down to her personality, which is a key component with people's dealings with my autism; or it could be her neuroscience training as autism is a neurological condition.

After graduating from Cambridge, Charlotte worked for a construction company named 8build in London from February 2012 until November 2013. However, during this time, she went to the pub rather than the gym after work. Without a goal, Charlotte found the gym boring and didn't see the point in, "sweating with a group of silent strangers in a spin class. It felt just weird."

At this juncture, Charlotte founded *Rabble* along with Rosemary Pringle, who now lives in Australia. It is a business that "extols the virtues of getting fit by having fun." Charlotte wanted to meet up with "a group, at a time that suited, and do something active and fun."

Rabble started in January 2014, as Charlotte ploughed her life savings into the business and "lived off fear." Initially, events were free, to gauge popularity, as Charlotte posted on the social network meetup.com to ask if anyone wanted to "play schoolyard games in London."

Following this, certain angel investors and Downing Enterprises of Cambridge University invested £210,000. Cambridge Angels chairman, John Yeomans, said he was "blown away" as they usually only invest in tech start-ups. It looks like their investments will be rewarded as Rabble is on track to make their first profit in 2017.

Although Charlotte explained to me that she is now "an anti-elite level advocate" she also feels that the elite level is "one-dimensional" and "sucks the fun out of training whilst losing sight of the enjoyment of exercise."

After meeting Charlotte, and hearing topical stories of the "win at all costs" attitude of British Cycling and Team Sky (encapsulated by the Jess Varnish "saga" and the treatment she is said to have received), her approach certainly resonated with me. At times, even as a spectator, you wonder if it is really worth all that mental, physical and emotional intensity just to win. Perhaps it was more fun in the past, both as a viewer and competitor, when athletes in all elite level sports seemed to have a better-rounded view of life. Many of them had other jobs. England cricket's record test scorer, Alastair Cook, for example, seems to have a well-rounded view of his job; when he is not playing cricket, he works on his smallholding farm with wife, Alice.

Fortunately, Charlotte, like myself, and millions around the U.K., can enjoy exercise in a fun environment whilst bringing the best out of us mentally, emotionally and physically. This is why Charlotte started Rabble – to make things as fun as possible.

Charlotte loved the different games of P.E. as a child, and wanted a "playground scenario" to take shape with Rabble. I told Charlotte of the lack of support that my niece – Chloe – had received at her school with P.E., which had put her off exercising, and what (we felt) were "box ticking exercises" regarding the teaching of the subject. Charlotte told me that this was "short-sighted" and that it is the school's job to "engage people to try to get them participating in exercise." As she explained, "People thrive in spite of the schools… schools don't focus on general health which could be life-changing." She also thinks, "School should create good patterns for life, but they end up having the opposite effect with people catching up decades later."

The rules to Rabble are "flexible" and it helps "people forget" they are even exercising, although they have to move "a lot" to win. According to Charlotte, "Exercise is just movement" and "there are so many ways to move." Charlotte's mother, Chris, takes the sessions in Chester, which started in March 2016, and is the oldest to take part at age 58. Typically, the age range is between 20 and 40.

There are over 500 varied games in the Rabble cannon with two types of difficulty. It costs £7 a week for membership, although "newbies" are invited to three complimentary sessions to help "inactive people" get exercising.

Rabble has now spread to Manchester, Chester, Liverpool, Cambridge, Sheffield, Edinburgh, Nottingham, Brighton and Bristol. To further the social aspect, Charlotte wanted to build a "socially diverse community" that offered "a supportive environment." There are black tie events, camping in the Peak District, special occasion events (like celebrating Halloween), and more. In fact, the day after I met Charlotte, there was a Rabble derby taking place between Chester and Manchester (Manchester won all the ball games including circular dodgeball).

Charlotte's future plans are very interesting and quite intriguing. These include using games to help 'referred' people to exercise. As Charlotte asked me, "How many referrals stay?" and the answer is not very many (which goes to show the 71% that Rochdale Mind retained, in the last quarter of 2016, to be a very impressive statistic). Charlotte's plan regarding this is to use "games for referred patients to have fun rather than being told to do it."

In addition to this, Charlotte is working on getting 16-25-year-old mental health patients, in the South East of England, to join "one or two sessions a week to build confidence" which she hopes will end up in "group forming." Charlotte also hopes to work with the Refugee Council to "open spaces at sessions specifically for refugees." In my opinion, it is lovely to see someone with a social conscience regarding people who are less fortunate.

After reading the back of my memoirs, Charlotte kindly decided to buy a copy of

"I've Got a Stat For You" there and then. Furthermore, as we parted, she left me with some very wise words of wisdom. For, you see, I had told her that I struggled after the goal of writing my memoirs was complete. After I was published, I felt empty since a big ambition in my life had been achieved. Charlotte concurred, "When you had the goal of writing your memoirs, it drove you on. Achievement doesn't feel as big and you can feel hollow."

All in all, I found Charlotte to be an extremely engaging young woman with an infectious personality. I would delighted to bump into her again in the future. I hesitate to use this word, but I wish this *inspirational*, yet engaging and socially conscious lady, all the best in her future success.

12. Rosie Henry

Whilst perusing the BBC News application, as part of my usual early morning routine towards the end of my book research in October 2017, I came across a very interesting story about a female powerlifter. I am currently training for a powerlifting competition myself, and the report on her backstory grabbed my attention instantly.

The lady's name was Rosie Henry, a 40-year-old from Falmouth in Cornwall. Reading her story, online, I was struck by the many physical and emotional obstacles she had overcome or managed. So with this in mind, I managed to contact Rosie via Fitness Wild, a company which runs outdoor, personal fitness sessions and a female powerlifting club.

Firstly, I asked Rosie about the many and varied challenges that she has overcome.

"I feel if I were to write down every mental and physical battle I have had to overcome, it would be a book in itself. I can almost talk about myself in the third person, as it often seems that it was someone else's life I was experiencing. I think, in a way, to detach myself from the experiences was the only way I could survive them. There are people out there who have been through much, much worse, or much less – but it does not diminish your own personal anguish, as your struggles are unique to you.

"I do not feel, at this juncture, it is right for me to trawl back too deep, too much into the past. However, as a teenager I went through my own difficulties of depression, eating disorders, and chronic fatigue while suffering from glandular fever. Also, I suffered a sexual assault which led to me testifying against my perpetrator, and another hospitalisation after I had my drink spiked. In addition to this, I was in an abusive marriage, as well as undergoing a series of operations on my hip. I came through all this relatively unscathed, I thought, and had a happy period having moved back to the UK from America, after meeting my partner while forging a successful career.

"In my thirties, following the birth of my son, Oscar, I discovered I had bone degeneration in my neck which nerve conduction tests confirmed. I had lost feeling in parts of my body. The pain was agonising, and there were some days I couldn't even hold my son. I was looking into having surgery when I found out I was unexpectedly expecting my second child. Surgery had to wait. Meg came along as Oscar turned 15 months.

"I was living in a county where I knew no one, and we had no support, and I think this is how my post-natal depression took hold so fast and so strongly. It was a quick spiral downwards, and I was referred to the supervision of the psychiatric team. I honestly believe I had reached such depths of depression that my body gave up. I contracted viral meningitis which let to my first hospitalisation for ten days and then, a couple of months after – still not feeling well – I succumbed to an infection which led me to go into respiratory before suffering a cardiac arrest. I truly believe it was only through my body failing and then being given this second chance that I was able to overcome my mental health battles and start on my journey to wellness."

Following her eventful past, Rosie moved to Falmouth in 2012 where she opened a coffee shop before linking up with Fitness Wild, which is based at Argal Reservoir and Gyllyngvase Beach. I asked Rosie what prompted her to move to Cornwall to start a new life and new career.

"The tipping point was finding out I was pregnant in my mid-thirties. I suddenly felt trapped in my corporate life, in a hamster wheel of flights and meetings with long hour days. I realised I didn't want to be the mum trying to juggle it all and accomplishing nothing. With the support of my partner, we decided – almost on a whim – to move to Cornwall. It seemed crazy at the time to give up a successful career and financial security, but we did it. We moved to Cornwall. The first two years were a blur of mental fog, illness and being a mum to two young children. The next two years were about me getting well, and the last year has been about my transition to a healthy person and investing in the people who saved me. I had been attending Fitness Wild classes for my whole period of rehabilitation. I then got to a point where I knew I could take on and do more. My little girl was starting school and I knew I would have the time to give back something. A café, which is called Wild Vibes, came up for sale locally and we knew, in conjunction with Fitness Wild, it would make a perfect HQ for the growth of the company."

I then moved onto the subject of powerlifting, as someone who is entering their first novice powerlifting competition soon. I asked Rosie what first attracted her to training for the sport.

"I never intentionally went into powerlifting. Two years ago, I went into training not being able to do a squat or stand on one leg, so the thought of 'lifting' was never there. As I got stronger, though, I realised I had an innate strength and determination. My trainers believed in me, and for once I did too. I signed up for my first competition in November 2017, more to encourage other women to do so. For them to not feel any pressure or anxiety but see it as a step to self-fulfilment and empowerment.

"I never expected to win. So to find out I have automatically qualified for the British drug-free championships in February 2018 is something of a shock!"

Having changed trainers in April 2017, after a bad experience, I found that I enjoyed training more than ever and I wondered whether Rosie could explain the buzz she gets from powerlifting.

"It is almost like a form of meditation for me. I find it is the one thing I can solely focus on. It's just the bar and me. A lot of sport is down to mind over matter, your mind limits what your body can achieve, and by just believing in yourself, you are halfway there to making it possible.

"Unlike other sports, it is truly about you. All your fellow competitors want to see you achieve as much as you want them to. There is a real sense of camaraderie and support I've never found in any other competitive sport.

"Plus I do it outside; sun, wind, or rain I train. Being out in the elements is so primal; it's where our bodies are meant to be, not stuck at a desk 24/7. Your soul thanks you for it. Personally, I could never now do a sport if it meant I couldn't train outside."

Apart from powerlifting, I wondered which sports Rosie attempted previously, between her physical and emotional battles. She told me, "To be honest after coming out of hospital, my body was so weak it's no wonder everything I tried I failed at – dance classes, running groups, going to the gym. I wasn't listening to my body.

"Yoga massively helped with my emotions and learning to be more still and mindful, but I needed to feel strong too. My mantra became: if I can't be mentally strong, I'm damn well going to get as physically strong as I can. This would never have happened if I hadn't met FW. They literally went back to basics on how I stood, sat, walked and we did a year-and-a-half of small tiny exercises over and over again, rebuilding me. It was not a quick fix. It was a fundamental life change."

I asked what Rosie's expectations where upon entering a competition. I told her that my coach, Geraint, informed me that you are competing against yourself to achieve the best of your potential.

"I have no expectations – hand on heart. I am not going to win it, but I go for the experience, for being part of something, to support my fellow athletes. Two years ago, I would never have thought competing would have been possible! I'm honoured to be alive and to be standing in front of my children showing that, if you try hard enough, you can accomplish anything.

Rosie then elaborated further to explain how powerlifting contest categories work.

"The competition is split into age categories, (I compete in Masters1 as I am over 40) and also weight categories, so you compete with similar strength people. We are all different in the world, we are all different shapes and sizes, and we don't judge. All our bodies can do AMAZING things and we should respect it and others."

I asked Rosie what her advice would be to anyone who may be thinking of training for powerlifting and why she thinks it is such a great sport to take up. Personally, I like the fact that it is about gym fitness and skills rather than needing to have a great natural ability that would be required in most sports. Literally, anyone who trains hard to a decent standard with great technique can get involved; it also focuses on what you can do rather than what you can't achieve.

"There are SO many reasons powerlifting is good for you. I wouldn't know where to start! Strength is one of the most important things you can give yourself. Most people assume cardio equates with good overall training. However, training for strength and conditioning is much more beneficial.

"In my opinion, there are ten commonly identified aspects of fitness which are:

1. Cardiac/respiratory endurance
2. Stamina
3. Strength
4. Flexibility
5. Power
6. Coordination
7. Speed
8. Agility
9. Balance
10. Accuracy

"Of these ten aspects, strength and conditioning effects all ten whilst having a significant impact on nine. Cardio endurance work leads to very specific changes that are, in my opinion, not long-term. Whereas the effects of strength and conditioning training gives stronger muscles, improved bone density and thick tendons; they are long-lasting and slow the progression of aging and greatly improve your quality of life – mentally and physically.

"What's not to love?!"

Finally, I asked Rosie what the best advice she had received in life or training was.

"There are so many cliché life platitudes. The most difficult paths in life lead you to amazing destinations, "believe and you will achieve," "this too shall pass."

"Life is in my control. How I react to it, and whatever it throws at me in the future, it is going to be ok because I have that belief in myself – I've got this."

After hearing Rosie's interesting, varied, and inspirational life, the reasons I started to write this book were reinforced. I wanted to find the incredible people that masquerade as everyday people. It seems to me that there are more interesting stories from "regular" people rather than the vacuous human beings who pervade our television screens on so-called reality television. These are the people that should be on prime time, rather than those on *TOWIE* or *I'm A Celebrity Get Me Out of Here*, *Strictly Come Dancing* or *The X- Factor*. The people in this book are, in my opinion, the real stars.

13. Lord's Taverners

In the midst of "The Calypso Summer" of 1950 that saw "those two little pals of mine Ramadhin and Valentine" rip through England at Lord's to seal the West Indies' first ever Test cricket win in England (on their way to a 3-1 series win), a charity with cricket and philanthropy at its core was founded to raise funds for worthwhile and needy causes.

The Lord's Taverners was founded on the 3rd of July 1950 by cricketers from the acting profession with Martin Boddey as its chair. The club launched in the Circle Bar of the Comedy Theatre, and 71 members signed up for its first meeting on the 2nd of September 1950, including the legendary Jack Hobbs, who was the first professional cricketer to be knighted (in 1953). This was 27 years after Francis Eden Lacey was knighted for his 28 years as MCC Secretary.

Within the first year of the charity's foundation, an eclectic mix of acting, broadcasting, and cricketing personalities had become members, with well-known personalities a feature of the charity's public promotional work to this day. In turn, the presidents of the charity reads like a who's who of showbiz, royalty, and cricket; they include three former England captains and three members of the Royal Family with literally a whole host of acting and television "A-listers" as well. Sir John Mills became the first President in 1950.

The first recipient of the charity's generosity was the National Playing Fields Association, who were the sole beneficiaries for the first 15 years of The Lord's Taverners with donations mostly used for the installation of artificial cricket wickets.

Nowadays, the fundraising and charity work branches out far and wide with £3.4m spent on funding equipment, facilities, programmes and resources (2016 figures). Indeed, of that sum, 43.4% was spent on securing 40 minibuses, 18.5% on disability cricket, 14.5% on indoor and outdoor equipment, 12% on community cricket, 9% on junior sports development, and 2.6% on recycling sports kit.

Amongst the £3.4m spent on charitable and needy causes were 23 sensory rooms, which can be used by people with Autistic Spectrum Condition amongst others, seven outdoor play spaces, recycled kit sent to 13 different nations, and 77 multi-sport wheelchairs.

Fundraising events in 2016 included a Dinner for Wicketkeepers which saw some of the all-time Test wicketkeeping greats from several eras raise

£100,000, and a lunch with cricketing "jack of all trades" David "Bumble" Lloyd raise £60,000.

Twenty-five regions in the United Kingdom have a branch of The Lord's Taverners, whilst sister charities include The Sports Wheelchair Sponsorship Scheme launched in 2002 with Dame Tanni Grey-Thompson as its patron, and The Brian Johnston Trust. The latter awards scholarships to "those in need" and blind cricketers, with 22 handed out in 2016 to help with coaching, travel, and equipment. Over the last four years (until May 2017), The Brian Johnston Memorial Trust had funded 250 spin bowlers with 20 players already appearing for county first XI's.

Currently, the England and Wales Cricket Board are principal advisers on how funds by The Lord's Taverners are spent. Nonetheless, there are literally dozens of varied ways that the money is spent. This is most definitely the case with the sport of Boccia, which is a disability sport that has Paralympic status where players propel balls close to a target ball. There are two teams made up of either individuals, pairs, or a team of three over a set of ends. A ball can be thrown, rolled, or kicked. A ramp can be utilised for those unable to throw or kick. The Lord's Taverners run a nationwide under-19 tournament for Boccia.

Wheelchair Basketball is another supported sport. With 73 teams nationwide playing, including Under 15 and Under 19 national leagues, and a junior championship, The Lord's Taverners donate specially-adapted sports wheelchairs to disabled young people who require multi-sports starter chairs. Clubs of various sporting disciplines that cater for people with physical disabilities can apply for a maximum of five chairs.

Amongst those to have played wheelchair basketball, and who have benefitted greatly from the fundraising work of The Lord's Taverners, is Leanne Darrien. Leanne has seen her life transformed by the sport. Initially, she was only able to push one length of the court, but now has enough stamina to play two back-to-back matches totalling three hours. Leanne elaborated on her, and her fellow players, improvements to me.

"I have seen players brought completely out of their shells, showing sides of their personality – such as competitiveness – which those who do not understand their true capabilities have discouraged in the past.

"In giving me my own chair, The Lord's Taverners have been invaluable in my development and really made me feel part of a team."

In addition to Leanne, Gemma Lumsdaine of Dundee Dragons Wheelchair Basketball Club has seen enormous improvement from exercise and the work of The Lord's Taverners to promote an inclusive and healthy lifestyle with mental, physical and emotional wellbeing at its core. Gemma elaborated:

"The Lords Taverners Basketball Junior Championships and Junior League have had a massive impact on my life. Being able to compete and socialise with other young people with a disability has helped me develop my self-confidence and improve my self-esteem.

"Without these competitions, I wouldn't have had the amazing opportunities which have made me the person I am today."

However, with Lord's in the title of the charity, it is hardly surprising that cricket-based activities make up a fair amount of The Taverners' work. With the increased profile, media coverage, and money that has come into the women's game in recent years, it is interesting to note that almost half of the current England Ladies set-up have progressed through Under 11, 13 and 15 tournaments run by The Lord's Taverners. Amongst those to have come through are current captain Heather Knight, Anya Shrubsole, and wicketkeeper Sarah Taylor.

Each year, The Lord's Taverners run national tournaments for young girl cricketers. In 2016, these were won by Hazelgrove School of Somerset at Under 13 level and Ormskirk School from Lancashire at Under 15. In The Lady Taverners Girls National T20 finals, held at Grantham CC in Lincolnshire, the spoils went to J&G Meakin (Under 13) and North Devon CC (Under 15).

One cricket-based programme run by The Lord's Taverners that aims to help rid Britain of childhood poverty in lower income areas, especially those with a lack of accessible and "high-quality" clubs and facilities in their locale, is *Wicketz*.

Statistically, there are said to be 3.7m children in the United Kingdom living in poverty which equates to 28% of the childhood population. To attract its core target demographic of children from lower-income families, sessions are totally free.

Wicketz attempts to use the power of cricket as a tool for change, social cohesion, and to make a difference to people's lives in deprived areas. A "robust" mapping exercise of the United Kingdom identified the 20 most deprived areas with a desire to participate in cricket. Initially, West Ham and Tower Hamlets in East London were used as pilot areas with the programme subsequently spreading to Luton and Hartlepool. Further projects have been outlined for the future in Birmingham, Bristol, Nottingham, Sussex, and Plymouth.

Statistically, less than five percent of youngsters join "traditional" cricket clubs with disadvantaged areas said to have 40% less engagement in sport overall. Wicketz believes that young people, irrespective of background and ability, should have the chance to play cricket whilst taking part in physical activity.

One of Wicketz' success stories is 16-year-old Abdus Salaam from Luton. Although Abdus has only been playing for less than a year, he is an integral part of Luton Wicketz Club. Abdus witnessed domestic abuse in his early life, which led to him displaying severe anger management issues. He was tempted to "take the wrong path."

Fortunately, he was introduced to sport as a way to overcome and positively manage his emotions but also to diffuse arguments with others and develop sensitivity and maturity. Abdus explained, "I faced a few challenges in my upbringing and sport has really helped me out; you see a lot of kids growing up in Luton doing the wrong things and I'm happy that Wicketz has come to Luton to inspire me and my friends to play cricket as there aren't many opportunities to play sport locally."

Abdus has encouraged his peers to join him on the cricket pitch rather than follow a path of anti-social behaviour. He was rewarded for this by winning the Wicketz residential "Spirit of Cricket" award and the "Judge's Choice" at the Lord's Taverners Sporting Chance Awards.

The Lord's Taverners also run a disability cricket club. This is a year-round programme aimed at 14- to 25-year-olds that hosts over 2,000 coaching sessions, over the course of 12 months, of disability cricket to people with various disabilities. Based in London, by 2019 it is projected to cover all 32 boroughs of the capital.

One person to have greatly gained from the experience of being involved is Sam Alderson.

Sam has TAR Syndrome, a rare genetic disorder that is characterised by the absence of a radius bone in each forearm. Due to his condition, Sam thought his chances of playing cricket were over when he became a wheelchair user, but thanks to the LTDCC (Lord's Taverners Disability Cricket Club) it has given him a new lease of life.

After only two weeks of training with Bexley CC coach Dom Taylor, Sam's skills and self-confidence improved immeasurably. He began by playing in a powered chair but found being on his knees improved his game. He also found that due to only having two fingers on his hand, using a smaller bat was more comfortable and effective.

Sam still attended sessions at Bexley whilst he was injured and his infectious confidence helped his team-mates to better enjoy playing cricket and thus improve their performance. This resulted in Sam being named captain for the 2016 LTDCC Finals, where he won Most Improved Player. He later represented Kent Learning and Physically Disabled Team in the ECB Super Nines Tournament. Below are Sam's thoughts on his achievements and progression.

"I never thought I would be able to play cricket with my disability. When I became a wheelchair user, I thought it was gone for me and that I wouldn't be able to play sport again. I didn't know what to do, but luckily I was introduced to disability cricket and it has allowed me to once again experience all the excitement and happiness that sport gives me."

Grace Colverd is autistic and, like Sam, has seen disability cricket help her greatly. After returning to the U.K., after a period abroad, she was finding her feet at a new school and making new friends, which can be greatly challenging to put it mildly.

After starting sessions with Westminster Disability CC, Grace saw that being part of a team environment enabled her to make new friends, helped her social skills, and she learned how to communicate in a team with a shared kinship. Cricket has helped Grace settle into her new life more easily.

As well as traditional disability cricket, The Lord's Taverners offer the sport of Table Cricket. In 2016, there were 1,407 sessions of Table Cricket played under the auspices of the charity, with 19,458 participants.

You play table cricket with a paddle-like object acting as a bat, with defined areas representing fielding placements and run-scoring areas, and coaching sessions are offered to special education schools working with a range of disabilities to make the sport more inclusive. The national champions of table cricket are Ralph Thoresby School in Leeds. Dominic Nowland-Wall, a pupil at Ralph Thoresby School, explained his experiences of Table Cricket.

"I really enjoy table cricket. I like the training sessions and being part of a team. Table cricket has given me the opportunity to be actively involved in a sport for the first time in my life. Being in the winning team in the final at Lord's was the most wonderful achievement ever."

All in all, 1,042,765 sporting chances were offered in 2016 by The Lord's Taverners. From the evidence of this chapter, the charity has made an enormously positive impact on many people's lives. The charity has branched out far and wide during its almost 70-year existence and it is safe to say "They have made many hundreds of thousands of pals of their own" over this time whilst changing people's lives for the undoubted better. Here is to the next 70 years!.

Section 2

14. My Story

Due to my autism, I only relax when I am watching certain television programmes, like Great British Railway Journeys, or putting vinyl onto my iPod. In turn, once I had completed the writing of my first two books, I felt slightly lost with a different routine and less of a structure on a daily basis. After the release of the Brymbo Football and Cricket book, and I've Got a Stat for You - My Life with Autism, it felt as if I was coming off cloud nine.

I was missing something that didn't exist anymore.

On a daily basis, I became very nervous, agitated, snappy, antagonistic, lacking in confidence and struggling to cope with daily tasks that were hitherto accomplished. I was arguing with my family whilst bringing stress upon Mel – my sister – and Ma. My stress levels were very high and I was failing to bring them down. Meltdowns were becoming more frequent.

This lack of structure continued periodically for around 18 months and my autism reached boiling point with obsessional behaviours after a bad train trip back from London Euston after Joe Root's first test as England captain against South Africa. I won't burden you with the details but just to say I went on television to name and shame the train company, and got help from my regional Welsh Assembly member (who is Cross Party Autism Chair for Wales). Fortunately, this had a satisfactory conclusion, when I gave a presentation to the training staff of the company, who were very receptive, apologetic, and shocked at what had occurred.

Fortunately, this forced my hand and I had to find my own happiness. It prompted me to start volunteering, lifting very heavy objects like logs and stones at Wepre Park Country Park in Flintshire. The site is near to the River Wepre where The Stone Roses skimmed stones to create Breaking Into Heaven, the long 11-minute opening track off their 1994 LP The Second Coming. I also started volunteering for a local autism charity in Wrexham. I had to find my own happiness or I could have lost my freedom as my mental health had become that bad.

However, what helped me the most to overcome my stress was (and is) exercise. I was first introduced to the world of exercise at the turn of the millennium. This was when I started to support and follow Cefn Druids in the Welsh Premier League aged 15. As I had always struggled with my weight as a child, and indeed did when I was 15, for me it was very light exercise. For you see, although I was only a supporter of the Druids, I was allowed to join in twice-weekly training sessions where applicable.

It was around September 2000, ten months after first supporting Druids, that I started attending the gym. There was a brief flirtation, previously, when I was 12 when I went to a gym called Flex on the Wrexham Industrial Estate. After very light sessions in the gym, I plucked up the confidence to finally take part in P.E. sessions at St. Christopher's School.

During this time, I even had to build up to being able to run a mile without stopping around Alyn Waters Country Park in my home village of Gwersyllt in Wrexham. With my fitness improving, I even raised a few hundred pounds for my school, after arsonists had burned out the minibuses, and Druids (who were struggling financially at this juncture).

Unfortunately, in the autumn of 2003, I injured my knee and lost what little confidence I had gained. Although, even before the knee injury, I was quite overweight, I put more on during the winter of 2003-04 as, after leaving school, I was at a loose end a couple of days a week, as I only attended college for a day a week.

So, after visiting a physiotherapist, I decided to attend circuit training at a leisure centre in Wrexham. I was so unfit that I had to leave the class after 35 minutes due to being too tired. At this juncture, I was missing the buzz, badinage, camaraderie, and craic of the lads at Cefn Druids training sessions. These sessions had given me so much confidence and had helped my autism immensely. My social skills had developed with the lads, some of whom are still very close mates to this day. Being at Druids had given me a sense of belonging.

I continued to attend sessions of circuit training at my local gym but struggled at times with the big group of up to 60 people. If the instructor was different from the usual, it would freak me out and I would be antagonistic to the new instructor and not give them the respect they deserved. At times, on occasions of this nature, I would go home early as I could be quite inertly confrontational. It was all down to the change of routine, something that people with autism struggle greatly with.

I also attended sessions at other classes in North East Wales and Chester. Nonetheless, I still felt unfulfilled with these and as if I was just going through the motions of the workout. To combat this, I decided to take up weights and interval running with a programme printed from a website. With the running, I lost several stone and was the slimmest I will probably ever be, but I looked drawn and slightly older looking for it.

The running was the only relaxation in my day-to-day life, probably because I was too knackered to do anything else. At this time, I was struggling with clinical depression through changes in my working life and my behaviour was affected greatly due to my autism.

Although I lost weight from the running, and it had taken a slight amount of stress away from me, it was not what I wanted from training. I would always get stressed before my workouts, due to the sheer level of expectation I placed upon myself to achieve the best realistic results.

Also, at one point (not so long ago), if I was unable to train due to extreme weather like snow, or illness, I would be pacing around the house bemoaning the unforeseen situation that had arisen. Hitherto, I used to moan that I was going to gain weight and lose vast levels of conditioning. I had been told that I didn't give illness the respect it deserves. I wouldn't rest at the best of times, even when I was ill. I didn't sleep during the day or relax when I should.

After a great workout, I feel I have the power to tackle the stresses and strains of the rest of my day. The best way I can explain the feeling or sensation is by equating it to a person of religious faith who has attended their respective place of worship.

On the days I don't workout, I can frequently feel sluggish, lacking in zest, or trying to recreate the buzz and excitement I get from my workout. On these days, I can feel dopey, empty, and like I am missing a part of me.

Without exercise, my family, and my mates, I dread to think what would become of me. To people who claim they can't fit training into lives, I believe they are missing out on the biggest stress reliever of all. It gives me not only physical strength, but helps my mental and emotional state. Many of the lessons learnt from training can, in my opinion, help you think and act more clearly in life whilst aiding decision making processes.

All my thoughts on exercise over the years got me thinking. What are the positive experiences that other people must have had? And from that thinking, this book was born.

Unfortunately, in April 2017, my training had stagnated and I needed a fresh approach. I was no longer comfortable in my training environment. I also felt the training sessions had become far too predictable and I had put on a lot of weight due to the stress this was causing me with no nutritional advice forthcoming. I'd wanted to have a healthy diet for years, but due to a lack of education and over-complication from the trainers and instructors I'd encountered, I did not know how to eat well. I ate all the same foods in a very autistic manner. Fundamentally, I felt I needed a change and new approach.

My experiences have taught me that you must be comfortable in your environment. I've realised that I can't overemphasise this. I don't feel I had ever felt fully comfortable for a substantial period of time wherever I had trained up until this point. It was just so complicated. Surely it could be simpler?

I am proud to say that the setback of changing my trainers gave me the initiative to not be down for too long, and I looked forward to this new chapter of my training. My training sessions had become far too predictable, with the same six to eight exercises in each workout week in, week out. In fact, I recall the sense of dread I used to feel going to sessions in the months before I found Number One HSP and Geraint Roberts (more below).

Since training with Geraint at Number One HSP in April 2017, I have lost over three stone, got much fitter, stronger, healthier and athletic and I haven't EVER enjoyed my sessions anywhere nearly as much. In fact, before Geraint, I saw exercise as a necessity not an activity to be savoured and enjoyed. Geraint simplifies what could be complex information if delivered by someone else, and my autism is able to process it. He also encourages me greatly, whilst giving out clear, concise advice on how I could possibly improve my training and nutrition. Part of which is having an application called MyFitnessPal that collates and calculates all your calories and nutrients from over two million foods stored. Sorry for the advert! Geraint's motto is "There is more than one way to skin a cat," which takes into account that we are all individuals, whether you have autism or not.

Geraint also keeps sessions very fresh and extremely varied as I don't usually have a clue what is going to happen. In turn, Geraint creates a calm, stress-free environment that I feel extremely comfortable in. I seldom, possibly never, had experienced this before.

Geraint also keeps a record of every single exercise from every session since I joined to gauge my progress and to scientifically judge my continued performance. He also keeps the sessions fresh due to his continued appetite to learn well beyond his Masters in Sports Science/Strength and Conditioning with his undoubted desire to adapt and improve with the latest sports science research. He does this alongside Ed Harper, the founder and other day-to-day Director of Number One HSP alongside Geraint.

Due to Geraint's skill at training me, I entered a North West Powerlifting Event at UTC gym in Clatterbridge on the Wirral on Sunday 25th March 2018. The event was put back a week due to the weather front known as "The Beast From the East II." This was the culmination of many months planning and work from Geraint and me. On the day itself, I even broke a personal best in the deadlift and I also won a trophy! I couldn't have achieved any of this without Geraint. Thank you.

*

My sister and carer, Melanie, has an interesting story regarding her experiences with exercise and training. Her story is next...

15. Melanie's Tale

From seven months old, my daughter Chloe didn't sleep, so the only way I believed that I could function on a daily basis was by eating more to try to give myself the energy to cope through the day.

I didn't work as, at this point, Chloe had so many hospital appointments to attempt to find out why her muscles were so weak, why her sleep pattern was so disrupted, and why her behaviour was a struggle to deal with on a daily basis. Due to this, after taking Chloe and her brother Louis to school, I was in a zombie-like state all day as I was so tired.

In addition to this, Chloe had to go to bed at the same time every night, despite not sleeping, and it had to be after watching Peppa Pig on Nick Jr. She would have to complete this whole routine night after night. With all this, I had started to put on weight as I wasn't moving much during the day. I was so tired and not eating sensibly as I couldn't be bothered due to the exhaustion.

Chloe was finally diagnosed with Dyspraxia at age five. Getting the diagnosis was a nightmare and, as we experienced with my brother Andrew, there wasn't any help for child or family. My husband Billy worked long hours as Andrew's support worker and I was very lonely.

At this point, Andrew suggested I start going to the gym as I was complaining I was fat and unfit. Our mother, Hazel, offered to look after Chloe on a Monday evening, which was when Andrew went to circuit training.

Going to the gym was the best thing I have ever done. At first, I was really nervous and very self-conscious. I would quietly go to the gym and stay on the bike or just walk on the treadmill as I didn't have the confidence to run. I felt really good after each session and actually had more energy to cope better with life. Also, Mum worked really well with Chloe on a Monday evening and managed to change her routine which helped me immensely.

After five months of going to the gym, I decided to go to a Bodypump class with Andrew for the first time on Wednesday 9th December 2009. I was nervous but enjoyed the class. I carried on going to the gym on a Monday evening and to Bodypump on a Wednesday morning. I always felt alive and buzzing following these sessions. I coped so much better with life and Chloe's condition as, even though she didn't sleep well, I felt I had more energy due to exercising.

Around this time, I started to look at what I was eating and started to eat more healthily, and decided to start running on the roads when Chloe and Louis were in school. It helped clear my mind. I wasn't any good, but it greatly helped my mental health. I then decided to enter the BUPA Great Manchester 10km Run.

To prepare for the run, I ran three times a week, along with Bodypump and the gym. With hindsight, I believe I over-trained and lost too much weight. I completed the 10km in 69 minutes. I felt so emotional when I finished the run as I didn't think I'd complete something of this ilk. It felt good as I had achieved it for me.

I have since been able to complete the Delamere 10km Commando and the Duke of Edinburgh Diamond Challenge by walking up Scafell Pike and Snowdon, the highest peaks in England and Wales.

Although Chloe now sleeps and controls her condition infinitely better, I couldn't cope without exercise. I am now a full-time carer for Andrew, who is autistic, as all his funding was cut when he was made redundant. I love working with Andrew as it is very rewarding seeing what he has achieved, but it can, at times, be stressful. Exercise helps me copes with this stress.

I now incorporate the lessons learnt in exercise to everyday life as when Chloe was younger I didn't mix with people a lot. This really affected my confidence and self-esteem. It offers me a break from the family, including caring for Andrew.

In April 2017, as well as Andrew, my training sessions had unfortunately stagnated and, along with Andrew, I also started training at Number One Health Strength Performance. The facilities are fantastic with monkey bars, a rope climb, and a prowler sled amongst the strength and conditioning weights.

I love the fact that although the gym coaches a range of abilities, from elite athletes to myself, everyone that sets foot inside the gym is treated as an individual. The atmosphere is very friendly and relaxed with the coaches being really helpful; any questions you ask them are answered courteously and simply. When I am training, I feel I can ask questions without looking or feeling silly, or if I don't execute the correct form and technique on an exercise the first time around.

This, for me, is very important as I feel I can get the best out of my training when I am comfortable and relaxed in an environment of this ilk. This hasn't always been the case with some gyms I have attended in the past. When I feel confident and comfortable, I perform better. My coach

Geraint Llyr Roberts is fantastic. He is extremely educated in health, strength and conditioning.

Geraint also gave the simplified nutritional advice that Andrew and I had been craving for years by advising us to use an application called My Fitness Pal, which collates not just the calories, but all this within over two million foods, which of course is more than a human can store!

In a recent strength and conditioning challenge at the gym, I came second amongst the women and won protein supplements. I am entering a powerlifting competition in the near future. I looked up competition results in my weight category for an event in the North West of England for novices and was surprised to see that I was well on track to being better than some of the competitors.

As this book goes to print, I will be preparing to enter a North West powerlifting event in Manchester city centre in late April 2018. This will be the culmination of a year's hard work, and a vast improvement in strength and fitness levels; all due to the great coaching, calm understanding and planning of Geraint.

Like Andrew, exercise helps me deal with the stresses of everyday life. From a person who used to get breathless walking up the road with the severe asthma I suffered from across my childhood and through my twenties, to someone who can lift heavy weights and objects, execute exercises and run – the changes in me have been profound. I can now actually run a 10km in 52 minutes; that is 17 minutes quicker than when I ran the Great Manchester 10km in 2012.

I am now 45-years-old but there is no comparison to even when I was 20-years-old. I feel so much better about myself. Due to exercise, I feel a lot healthier, both mentally and physically. I wish I had found exercise years ago, but I wasn't ready. If I can do it, anyone can do it! There is no better feeling than the sense of achievement at the end of a session. I love it!

*

16. Number One Health Strength Performance

I have an enormous confession to make. For someone who has been talking up the virtues of physical exercise throughout this book, I realised a few months ago that, although I had been exercising since my late teens, I don't think I had actually enjoyed it. I saw it as a necessary evil for what I wanted.

Unfortunately, with my last trainer, we had reached an impasse and the relationship broke down of my accord after four years. At this point, I felt like giving it all up. On Thursday 13th April 2017, I spent hours online looking for trainers in North East Wales and Chester. By mid-afternoon, it wasn't looking good. I had spoken to around half a dozen trainers who didn't come close to meeting the set criteria I was looking for.

I had tried all manner of searches with all sorts of different keywords before I found a gym in Queensferry, Flintshire. The credentials of one of the trainers there met just about all of my criteria. So, at this stage, I picked up the telephone and rang the gym named Number One Health Strength Performance. I had nothing to lose at this stage, but couldn't begin to quantify what I was to gain.

The coach/trainer whose credentials I was so impressed by, online, answered the phone. We only talked briefly as he was with a client. He said he would ring back after the session. Rather at my wit's end at this juncture, I rang him back just after his session finished when we spoke in greater depth. He also spoke to my Ma, who goes on the phone in these situations to aid me; with my autism, I freeze up somewhat and don't always explain myself fully. We arranged to meet five days later for a consultation and to take a look around the gym.

From the moment I saw the facilities at Number One HSP, I was extremely impressed and knew I wanted to train there. I now train with Geraint Roberts Personal Training.

Geraint is a kind, polite, thoughtful, sweet and courteous lad. He gets his message across when he's training me calmly and conversationally which, in turn, makes me feel calm and clear. Technique and form are very important to Geraint, but he explains it so well that the message sinks in so quietly, concisely and clearly.

The facilities at Number One HSP are first class. There are monkey bars, a climbing rope, sleds with weights on, weight bags, ropes and, to quote the band Half Man Half Biscuit, "much, much more."

During my first five months, I lost around three stone (I had gained a lot of fat in the months leading up to going there at my old trainer).

With some issues arising with my autism in summer 2017, the only thing that kept me from doing something daft to myself or someone else was my sessions with Geraint. He has taken great pride in my physical development. My proudest gains are that I can now climb across a set of 21 monkey bars in 38 seconds, complete ten chin-ups on a bar (when I couldn't do any when I joined Geraint), execute pull-ups after every monkey bar, climb up a 30-foot rope, and I can push a prowler sled with 180kg of weight six metres in just 16 seconds.

So, with this book in mind, I decided to delve deeper into Geraint Llyr Roberts' opinions and ethos on health, fitness, strength and conditioning, as well as finding out more about how Number One Health Strength Performance opened as a non-profit, community-interest company in September 2015 with the founder and director Ed Harper.

25-year-old Geraint told me about what prompted him to go into his chosen career and about his background.

"I always wanted to work in the Sports industry. I had no real idea what exactly I would do, only that I wanted it to involve sports in some way, shape or form. As a boy, I played a variety of sports, including football, tennis, cricket, and golf.

"I studied Sports Science at Bangor University during 2011-2014 and attained a first-class degree (BSc Hons). My sports life became less prevalent during University as my social life took over! However, in my third year at Bangor, my friends and I set up a football team for the Welsh Society (Undeb Myfyrwyr Cymraeg Bangor), and we won the League Cup and came second in the league in our first season which we were very happy with!

"I proceeded to further my education by studying for a Masters Degree in Sports Sciences (Strength and Conditioning) at the University of Chester (2014-2015). During my time studying for my Masters, I worked with the senior rowing team (boys and girls) of King's School, Chester. This involved weekly gym sessions where I assisted in coaching as well as lab testing of the athletes. I was also given the opportunity to accompany the senior boys on their Easter training camp for a week in Ghent, where another student and I spent a lot of time measuring the athletes' urine samples... the not so glamorous side of working with a sports team!

"Following my Masters, I began working at Number One Health Strength Performance Gym in October 2015 and haven't looked back since! During my time at the gym, I have worked with a variety of athletes, including county-level swimmers, professional footballers, national level badminton players, and local netball and rugby teams. I currently work with Mold RUFC's Senior Men's team as a strength and conditioning coach. I also work with clients on a one-to-one basis at the gym, as well as coaching group classes at the gym."

30-year-old Ed Harper co-founded Number One Health Strength Performance, and graduated from Sheffield Hallam University with a BSc in Sports Science with Coaching, before attaining an MSc in Sport & Exercise Science: S&C / Physiology. He is a UK strength & conditioning accredited coach who has worked for an impressive array of professional and elite sports organisations including Sale Sharks, Wigan Warriors, the Welsh National Rugby League, The New Saints F.C. (the Football champions of Wales for the last seven seasons), The English Football Association, and the English Institute of Sport based in Sheffield, where many Team GB Olympians train in various sports.

Intrigued by the gym's formation and his ideas on training, I asked Ed, also a director of the gym, about the opening of Number One Health Strength Performance and how it began and evolved.

"The opening of the facility was a long process, from start to finish I think it took a little under two years. Originally, I was working out of a small council-owned facility leading a few open classes and supporting a few athletes every week. From this, I was able to build a small base of customers in the general public allowing me to build a reputation and identity within the community, meaning opening a larger facility was a relatively natural progression, although still a big jump!

"The best way to describe the not-for-profit aspect of the organisation is to think of it as exactly the same as a 'normal' business, as in we can still make a profit each year, and the goal is to maximise income. However, any profit that is made has to be channelled back into the business through designated streams e.g., community outreach, new equipment, facility restoration, etcetera."

Regarding training, Ed told me that, "Physical activity can come in all shapes and forms, from gym-based strength training to team sport and everything in between. Research has proven that all forms of physical activity can have a positive influence on an individual in a physiological or psychological capacity. Exercise creates a stimulus, meaning the body releases endorphins and hormones causing a change in the individual. Physically, the type of exercise (or stimulus) determines the body's reaction, e.g., muscular hypertrophy, strength, speed.

"Although, personally, I do not have vast experience in personal training, I have done some and worked with a few individuals but not extensively as a personal trainer or for any great period of time. My main experience lies in working with athletes predominantly in team sports. I have worked for professional rugby of both codes and football teams as well as international teams and athletes from a range of sports. Research has proven (and in my experience I believe it is clear) that the most efficient way for anyone to train is using the same basis as an elite athlete.

"By this, I mean I believe a far more effective way of achieving any physiological goal is to lift heavy and move well, rather than jumping from fad to fad like classes on trampolines or 'insanity.'"

Turning back to Geraint, I asked him about his beliefs and ethos on the mental, emotional and physical benefits that come with training. "Training is a great way to get rid of the stress of everyday life. Training gives you a distraction from whatever is going on in your life. It provides a feel-good factor because exercise leads to a release of endorphins throughout the body, which is why people (often) feel a sense of satisfaction following exercise! This association of happiness following exercise helps people to continue with training regimes because they know exercise will make them feel good and, as a result, they'll have positive health benefits such as lower stress levels, a better mental state of mind, healthier blood pressure and a reduced risk of cardiovascular disease to name a few; all of which help improve quality of life!

"I've seen many clients overcome their initial doubts regarding training and being pleasantly surprised with their personal successes in a relatively short time. Hard work and consistency are the main factors leading to success for clients and myself as a PT. The best training programme in the world won't work if an individual doesn't work hard during every training session. They need to treat their time outside of the gym as importantly as their time in the gym, as well, to achieve their goals, whatever they may be. There's no cookie cutter programme that will lead to success; training needs to become a part of your lifestyle if you want to succeed. The people that have had the most success are the people who realise this and adapt their lifestyle to suit their goals. By creating healthy habits, achieving their goals becomes much easier.

"Form during a given exercise is MUCH more important than the load lifted/moved during an exercise. Too many people become engrossed by how much weight they can lift; they put themselves at risk of serious injury for the sake of their ego. It's not big, and it's not clever. Thankfully, correct form is a vital part of our coaching practice at Number One Health

Strength Performance Gym because a healthy, pain-free body is a happy body!"

I then asked Ed and Geraint about the positive success stories they had encountered in their time working in the gym and from training elite level athletes. Firstly, Ed told me, "I recently supported the England Women's under 17 football team at the Euro finals in the Czech Republic. The team got to the last eight of the tournament from a very difficult position and a very tough qualifying group. Although the team did not win the tournament, the experience and opportunity were invaluable for the players as they continue their journey with the aim of making their senior debuts."

Furthermore, Geraint told me about other positive success stories he had encountered.

"I've had experiences of clients not being able to complete a single pull up/chin up, to then proceeding to perform multiple sets of pull-ups. Seeing clients achieve goals they once thought was impossible fills me with joy and it's one of the reasons I love what I do.

"I've had clients who initially came to me with lower back pain end up deadlifting multiple repetitions (reps) with more than 1.5 times their bodyweight on the bar, pain-free! Another struggled to complete one chin up; now in his second month of training with me, he can perform six chin-ups without resting!

"One of my clients, who's a team sport athlete (rugby union), has been recovering from an Anterior Cruciate Ligament (ACL) injury, and because of his injury, one of his legs (the injured leg) became a lot weaker than the other. This meant that his main lifts (i.e., squat and deadlift) were compromised as his stronger leg had to do more work to compensate for the weaker leg. Three months into his training programme, which involves plenty of bilateral (working two limbs at the same time) and unilateral (working one limb at a time) work, he's able to squat over 100kg and deadlift 140kg for multiple reps!

"A lot of people don't realise that as a PT, I do more than help people lose body fat and/or gain muscle mass. I help people to move pain-free, to recover from serious injuries and subsequently get even stronger than they were before by improving their strength, stability, and mobility, making them stronger, more robust athletes. This subsequently improves their quality of life, meaning they can continue to do the things they enjoy doing without worrying about previous injuries getting in the way."

Geraint elaborated further when I asked him about his tips to succeed in your training.

- Be consistent and persistent.

- Treat training and being healthy as a lifestyle choice, not a chore. Fitness shouldn't be a 'fad' you do for a couple of weeks at a time throughout the year; it should be a habit set for life.

- Set healthy, realistic and sustainable habits that will set you up for living a healthier, happier life. This means having to work out the logistics of how your training routine fits in and around your work schedule. Some people may have less time to train than others due to work or family commitments, but everyone can find some time to exercise during the day, whether it's a 15-minute High Intensity Training (HIT) session or a 1-hour resistance training session.

- Respect the fact that your body needs to rest and recover between training sessions to subsequently come back stronger. Your muscles get stronger when you're outside of the gym, not while you're in it!

Epilogue

I would like to take this opportunity to thank the following people who have contributed to this book along the way. I'm indebted to you all.

Firstly, great thanks and much appreciation to legendary England bat/wicket-keeper Sarah Taylor. It is great honour for me to have my favourite female cricketer – as well as four-time Ashes winner, and three-time World Cup winner over the two shorter formats – on board with my book.

Sarah's profile, public advocacy, bravery and candour in speaking out about her own personal struggles with some of the issues raised in this book made her a natural fit to write the foreword. Sorry I left it so late to ask you, Sarah, but when I should have asked you – at the Lancashire Thunder v Surrey Stars match at Old Trafford in August 2017 – I was having mental health issues of my own.

Thanks go, in chapter order, to:

Sabrina and Paula Fortune

Melanie Tilley from Rochdale Mind

Andrew Ruscoe from Brickfield Rangers F.C.

Ian Martin, Ben Walker, Ross Hunter & Martin Dean from the England & Wales Cricket Board

Henry Cowen (England Women's Media Manager) for putting me in contact with Sarah Taylor. He even called me from India to sort out my query!

England Visually Impaired Cricket Team

North Wales Crusaders Wheelchair Rugby League Club

Kris Saunders-Stowe at Wheely Good Fitness

Councillor Andrew Atkinson for driving me to Ross on-Wye!

Amy Webster from The National Autistic Society

Danby Rovers F.C.

Autism Plus, Sheffield

Andrea Smith at Cwm Wanderers F.C.

George Crewe and all at Wrexham Amateur Boxing Club

Joey Jones

Charlotte Roach MA (Hons) Cantab

Rosie Henry

Ana Hickey from The Lord's Taverners

Geraint Llyr Roberts MSc (Sports Sciences- Strength and Conditioning) & Ed Harper MSc Sport & Exercise Science: S&C / Physiology at Number One Health Strength Performance

James Lumsden-Cook from Bennion Kearny for allowing me to take this project on by agreeing to publish it before I undertook any work on the book, and it was only a very rough idea.

And last, but by no means least, my mother, Hazel Davies, and my sister/carer, Melanie Beckley for accompanying me, their help, support, the original idea from Mel of writing a book on this subject, and their general assistance.

My life has been a rollercoaster experience for me, both personally and professionally, since I got the all clear to write this tome in 2016.

Nonetheless, it has been an extremely enjoyable experience, especially when I have put my mind to it. Sometimes I have got waylaid both personally, emotionally and professionally, as there are so many stories out there. In fact, quite a few people turned down the opportunity to contribute to the book, but when I came to calculate the pages typed on my pen drive towards the end of the research process, I was ecstatic at how much information I had collated from the book's many, kind contributors.

Personally, the best lesson I have learned regarding exercise and training, during the writing of this book, is that you can achieve almost anything you put your mind to when you are in a comfortable environment and good space mentally. I can't overemphasise – if you are fortunate enough to be in a comfortable, encouraging environment – that you can challenge yourself mentally and physically in ways you never thought possible.

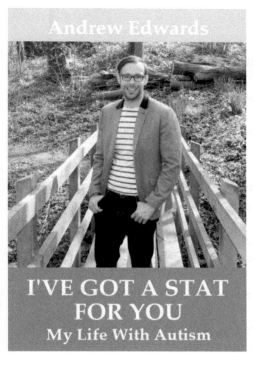

I've Got a Stat For You: My Life With Autism

By Andrew Edwards

At the age of four, Andrew Edwards was diagnosed with autism. "Go home and watch Rain Man," the specialist told his mother. "In all probability your son will be institutionalised." Determined to prove the specialist wrong, Andrew's mother set out to give her son the best life possible.

I've got a Stat for You is an honest and compelling account of one young man's journey to manage his autism and achieve his goals. Raised in a single parent household and encountering bureaucracy, bullying, and a lack of understanding from many around him, Andrew emerged from a turbulent childhood to win a Welsh National Young Volunteer Award, give speeches on his condition, and secure his dream job as a statistician at Manchester United Television.

From Wrexham to Buckingham Palace, and incorporating stories of The Simpsons, sport, music, and strange smells – *I've got a Stat for You* is a powerful and inspirational tale that shows how determination, a positive outlook, and the will to succeed can overcome all odds!

Testimonials

"Self-aware and very funny." **Stewart Lee**

"If you have a friend or relative with autism then this really is a must read." **Hayley McQueen, Sky Sports**

"Andrew's ability to fight against the odds is an inspiration to many others." **BBC Wales Today**

"A rare feat" **BBC Five Live Afternoon Edition**

"Fascinating" **John Humphrys, BBC Radio Four Today**

"Excellent insight into a very self-aware young Man with autism." **Book Nook**

"After reading his story, I have a better understanding of how our son connects things or people to certain events." **Beauty Brite Blog**

"This book is more than just autism. It is a families struggle to be heard in a world full of red tape." **Savette.com**

"This book shows how Andrew has shone through." **Talk Radio Europe**

"It is an interesting read and it makes one feel like you actually know the author and are part of his life." **Autismnow.com**

"This book is a true testament to determination and if you work hard and believe in yourself with the help of your family, you CAN do it." **Kellysthoughtsonthings.com Blog**

"Today, Andrew lives not just a normal, but indeed an exceptional life." **mom-spot.com**

"Absolutely a "must read" for anyone who lives or works with an autistic person- or for anyone interested not just in autism, but in the complexities of human communication." **Michellesblog.co.uk**

"Really interesting to read." **The Radcliffe and Maconie Show, BBC 6 Music**

"Offers a fascinating insight into the condition." **Welsh Daily Post**

"Andrew's family haven't had an easy life but they work so well as a team." **Daily Express Online**

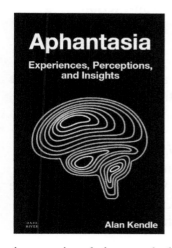

Aphantasia: Experiences, Perceptions, and Insights

by Alan Kendle

Close your eyes and picture a sunrise.

For the majority of people, the ability to visualize images – such as a sunrise – seems straightforward, and can be accomplished 'on demand'. But, for potentially some 2% of the population, conjuring up an image in one's mind's eye is not possible; attempts to visualize images just bring up darkness.

Although identified back in the 19th century, Aphantasia remained under the radar for more than a century, and it was not until recently that it has been rediscovered and re-examined. It has become clear that Aphantasia is a fascinating and often idiosyncratic condition, and typically more complex than the simple absence of an ability to visualize. People with the condition – Aphants – commonly report effects upon their abilities to recreate sounds, smells and touches as well; many also struggle with facial recognition. Paradoxically, many Aphants report that when they sleep, their dreams incorporate colour images, sound, and the other senses.

Put together by lead author Alan Kendle – who discovered his Aphantasia in 2016 – this title is a collection of insights from contributors across the world detailing their lives with the condition. It offers rich, diverse, and often amusing insights and experiences into Aphantasia's effects. For anyone who wishes to understand this most intriguing condition better, the book provides a wonderful and succinct starting point.

Foreword by Professor Adam Zeman, *Professor of Cognitive and Behavioural Neurology, University of Exeter*

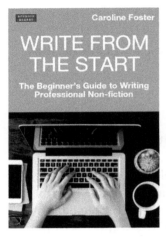

Write From The Start: The Beginner's Guide to Writing Professional Non-Fiction

by Caroline Foster

Do you want to become a writer? Would you like to earn money from writing? Do you know where to begin?

Help is at hand with *Write From The Start* – a practical must-read resource for newcomers to the world of non-fiction writing. It is a vast genre that encompasses books, newspaper and magazine articles, press releases, business copy, the web, blogging, and much more besides.

Jam-packed with great advice, the book is aimed at novice writers, hobbyist writers, or those considering a full-time writing career, and offers a comprehensive guide to help you plan, prepare, and professionally submit your non-fiction work. It is designed to get you up-and-running fast.

Write From The Start will teach you how to explore topic areas methodically, tailor content for different audiences, and create compelling copy. It will teach you which writing styles work best for specific publications, how to improve your chances of securing both commissioned and uncommissioned work, how to build a portfolio that gets results, and how to take that book idea all the way to publication.

Comprised of 16 chapters, there is information on conducting effective research, book submissions, writing for business, copyright and plagiarism pitfalls, formatting, professional support networks, contracts and agreements, the value of humour, ghostwriting, and much more…

By the end of this book – full of practical advice and proven results – you will be well on your path to writing success!

Lightning Source UK Ltd.
Milton Keynes UK
UKHW052302090219
336962UK00009B/160/P